IAGES
**Recent Advances in
Minimal Access Surgery-3**
(Robotic & Innovative Technologies)

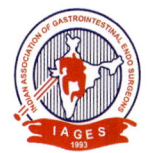

IAGES
Recent Advances in
Minimal Access Surgery-3
(Robotic & Innovative Technologies)

Editor-in-Chief

Subhash Khanna
MS FRCS (Edin) FICS FIAGES (Hony) FALS (Hony) FICLS (Hony) FAGIE
Founding President, Association of Robotic and Innovative Surgeons
Trustee, Indian Association of Gastrointestinal Endo Surgeons
International Academic Co-ordinator, Indian Association of Gastrointestinal Endo Surgeons
Vice President, International College of Surgeons (Indian Section)
Honorary Visiting Professor, Department of Surgical Gastroenterology
GSL Medical College, Rajahmundry, Andhra Pradesh
Dean, Swagat Academy of Medical Sciences
Chief Medical Director and Chief Consultant, Swagat Endolaparoscopic Surgical
Research Institute and Swagat Super Specialty Surgical Institute
Editor-in-Chief, Recent Advances in Minimal Access Surgery
President, Indian Association of Gastrointestinal Endo Surgeons (2018–19)
Convener Fellowship Board-IAGES (2016)
Ex-Vice President, Hernia Society of India
Ex-Governing Council Member, Association of Surgeons of India (Assam Chapter)
Shantipur, Guwahati, Assam, India

Associate Editors

Pawanindra Lal
Director and Professor
Moulana Azad Medical College
New Delhi, India

M Kanagavel
Chairman
Association of Surgeons of India
(Tamil Nadu Chapter)

Invited Joint Editors

Sunil D Popat
Immediate Past President, IAGES

Ramesh Agarwalla
Trustee, IAGES

Chelliah Selvasekar
Consultant Colorectal and Laparoscopic
Surgeon, The Christie NHS Foundation Trust
Manchester, United Kingdom

Forewords
Barry Salky
Davide Lomanto

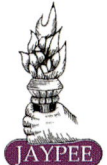

JAYPEE BROTHERS MEDICAL PUBLISHERS
The Health Sciences Publisher
New Delhi | London

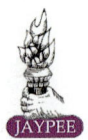 **Jaypee Brothers Medical Publishers (P) Ltd**

Headquarters
Jaypee Brothers Medical Publishers (P) Ltd
EMCA House, 23/23-B
Ansari Road, Daryaganj
New Delhi 110 002, India
Landline: +91-11-23272143, +91-11-23272703
+91-11-23282021, +91-11-23245672
Email: jaypee@jaypeebrothers.com

Corporate Office
Jaypee Brothers Medical Publishers (P) Ltd
4838/24, Ansari Road, Daryaganj
New Delhi 110 002, India
Phone: +91-11-43574357
Fax: +91-11-43574314
Email: jaypee@jaypeebrothers.com

Overseas Office
JP Medical Ltd
83 Victoria Street, London
SW1H 0HW (UK)
Phone: +44 20 3170 8910
Fax: +44 (0)20 3008 6180
Email: info@jpmedpub.com

Website: www.jaypeebrothers.com
Website: www.jaypeedigital.com

© 2023, Jaypee Brothers Medical Publishers

The views and opinions expressed in this book are solely those of the original contributor(s)/author(s) and do not necessarily represent those of editor(s) or publisher of the book.

All rights reserved. No part of this publication may be reproduced, stored or transmitted in any form or by any means, electronic, mechanical, photocopying, recording or otherwise, without the prior permission in writing of the publishers.

All brand names and product names used in this book are trade names, service marks, trademarks or registered trademarks of their respective owners. The publisher is not associated with any product or vendor mentioned in this book.

Medical knowledge and practice change constantly. This book is designed to provide accurate, authoritative information about the subject matter in question. However, readers are advised to check the most current information available on procedures included and check information from the manufacturer of each product to be administered, to verify the recommended dose, formula, method and duration of administration, adverse effects and contraindications. It is the responsibility of the practitioner to take all appropriate safety precautions. Neither the publisher nor the author(s)/editor(s) assume any liability for any injury and/or damage to persons or property arising from or related to use of material in this book.

This book is sold on the understanding that the publisher is not engaged in providing professional medical services. If such advice or services are required, the services of a competent medical professional should be sought.

Every effort has been made where necessary to contact holders of copyright to obtain permission to reproduce copyright material. If any have been inadvertently overlooked, the publisher will be pleased to make the necessary arrangements at the first opportunity.

Inquiries for bulk sales may be solicited at: jaypee@jaypeebrothers.com

IAGES Recent Advances in Minimal Access Surgery-3 (Robotic & Innovative Technologies)

First Edition: **2023**

ISBN: 978-93-5465-962-1

Printed at: Samrat Offset Pvt. Ltd

Dedicated to

*My mentor Late Prof B Dawka, for showing me how to take risks.
My wife Prof Swagata, for supporting me in pursuing my dreams
and helping convert into reality.*

Contributors

Ahmed Pervez MS MChEng
Registrar, Colorectal Surgery
The Royal Oldham Hospital
NCA NHS Foundation Trust
Manchester, United Kingdom

Amaniel Kefleyesus
Fellow
Department of Visceral Surgery
Centre Hospitalier Universitaire
Vaudois (CHUV)
Lausanne, Switzerland

Amay Banker MS
Senior Resident
Department of Surgery
KEM Hospital
Mumbai, Maharashtra, India

Amir Mushtaq Parray
Consultant
Department of Surgical
Gastroenterology, Bariatric and
Minimal Access Surgery
BLK-Max Super Specialty Hospital
New Delhi, India

Arun Kumar MS MCh
Fellow, Bariatric and Metabolic Surgery
Department of Surgical Disciplines
All India Institute of Medical Sciences
New Delhi, India

Arun Prasad MS FRCS FACS
Clinical Lead, Adjunct Professor,
Academic Advisor and Clinical Tutor
Department of GI, Bariatric and
Robotic Surgery
Indraprastha Apollo Hospital
New Delhi, India

Bana Rupa
Consultant
Department of Gynecology
Apollo Health City
Hyderabad, Telangana, India

Chelliah Selvasekar MD FRCS Ed MBA
Consultant Colorectal and
Laparoscopic Surgeon
Associate Medical Director of Clinical
Services and Specialist Surgery
Clinical Director
Manchester Surgical Skills and
Simulation Centre
The Christie NHS Foundation Trust
Manchester, United Kingdom

Deep Goel FACS (USA) FRCS (England)
Senior Director and HOD
Consultant Robotic Surgeon
Department of Gastro, Onco, Bariatric
and Advance Minimal Access Surgery
BLK-Super Specialty Hospital
New Delhi, India

Fabian Grass
Consultant Surgeon
Department of Visceral Surgery
Centre Hospitalier Universitaire
Vaudois (CHUV)
Lausanne, Switzerland

Gursev Sandlas MBBS MS MCh
(Pediatric Surgery) FAIS DHA FMAS
Consultant Pediatric Surgeon
Jaslok Hospital and Research Centre
Surya Children's Hospital
Mumbai, Maharashtra, India

Hugo Teixeira Farinha
Surgeon
Department of Visceral Surgery
Centre Hospitalier Universitaire
Vaudois (CHUV)
Lausanne, Switzerland

Jignesh Gandhi MS DNB FMAS FIAGES
DLS (France) Robotic Surgery (USA)
Professor
Laparoscopic and GI Surgeon
Department of Surgery
KEM Hospital
Mumbai, Maharashtra, India

Contributors

Kalpana Nagpal MS(ENT) DNB(ENT)
Senior Consultant and Robotic Surgeon
Department of ENT Head and Neck Surgery
Indraprastha Apollo Hospitals
New Delhi, India

Kalyan Pandey MCh
Surgical Oncology
Fellow in Robotic Surgical Oncology
Department of Oncosurgery
Manipal Hospitals
Bengaluru, Karnataka, India

Mamtha Reddy
Fellow
Department of Gynecology
Apollo Health City
Hyderabad, Telangana, India

Martin Hübner
Professor
Department of Visceral Surgery
Centre Hospitalier Universitaire Vaudois (CHUV)
Lausanne, Switzerland

Masafumi Inomata
Professor
Department of Gastroenterological and Pediatric Surgery
Oita University Faculty of Medicine
Oita, Japan

Matthew Boal
Research Fellow
Department of Surgery
General Surgery
Griffin Institute, United Kingdom

Nader Francis MBChB FRCS
Consultant Colorectal Surgeon
Yeovil District Hospital
NHS Foundation Trust
England, United Kingdom

Prasanna Ramana MS
Senior Resident (Academic)
Department of Surgical Disciplines
All India Institute of Medical Sciences
New Delhi, India

Raj Nagarkar MD
Professor and Chief of Surgical Oncology and Robotic Services
HCG Manavata Cancer Centres
Nasik, Maharashtra, India

Ravindra Vats
Senior Consultant
Department of Surgical Gastroenterology, Bariatric and Minimal Access Surgery
BLK-Max Super Specialty Hospital
New Delhi, India

Rooma Sinha
MD DNB MNAMS FICOG
Senior Consultant
Department of Gynecology
Apollo Health City
Hyderabad, Telangana, India

Sandeep Aggarwal MS FACS
Professor of Surgery
Department of Surgical Disciplines
All India Institute of Medical Sciences
New Delhi, India

Seigo Kitano MD
President and Professor
Department of Surgery
Oita University
Oita, Japan

Shyamanta M Hazarika
BE M Tech PhD
Professor and INAE
Abdul Kalam Technology Innovation National Fellow
Biomimetic Robotics and Artificial Intelligence Lab
Mechanical Engineering
Indian Institute of Technology Guwahati
Guwahati, Assam, India

Subhash Khanna MS FRCS (Edin) FICS FIAGES (Hony) FALS (Hony) FICLS (Hony) FAGIE
Founding President, Association of Robotic and Innovative Surgeons
Trustee, Indian Association of Gastrointestinal Endo Surgeons
International Academic Co-ordinator, Indian Association of Gastrointestinal Endo Surgeons
Vice President, International College of Surgeons (Indian Section)
Honorary Visiting Professor
Department of Surgical Gastroenterology
GSL Medical College
Rajahmundry, Andhra Pradesh
Dean, Swagat Academy of Medical Sciences
Chief Medical Director and Chief Consultant
Swagat Endolaparoscopic Surgical Research Institute and Swagat Super Specialty Surgical Institute
Editor-in-Chief, Recent Advances in Minimal Access Surgery
President, Indian Association of Gastrointestinal Endo Surgeons (2018–19)
Convener Fellowship Board-IAGES (2016)
Ex-Vice President, Hernia Society of India
Ex-Governing Council Member
Association of Surgeons of India (Assam Chapter)
Shantipur, Guwahati, Assam, India

Vitish Singla MS MCh
Senior Resident (Academic)
Department of Surgical Disciplines
All India Institute of Medical Sciences
New Delhi, India

Yasam Venkata Ramesh
MPharm PGDRA PGDBI PhD
Medical Writer
HCG Manavata Cancer Hospitals
Nashik, Maharashtra, India

Yohei Kono
Assistant Professor
Department of Gastroenterological and Pediatric Surgery
Oita University Faculty of Medicine
Oita, Japan

Foreword

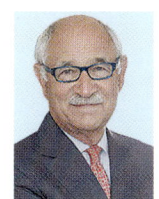

It is hard to believe that laparoscopic cholecystectomy began only about 35 years ago. Talk about disruptive technology in the field of surgery; It was clear then as it is now, that disruptive advances in laparoscopic surgery will continue. This third edition of "Recent Advances in Minimally Access Surgery" by IAGES, edited by Subhash Khanna, embraces this continuum by chapters on robotic surgery and other innovations. Almost since the beginnings of laparoscopic surgery, IAGES has been at the forefront of clinical advances in surgery, and it has been teaching it to others around the world from the start. This edition continues to awe and inspire colleagues practicing minimally access surgery. It is a must read for keeping up in our field, and maybe, a glimpse into the future.

Barry Salky MD FACS
Chief (Emeritus)
Division of Laparoscopic Surgery
Professor (Emeritus)
Department of Surgery
Mount Sinai Health System
New York City, New York, USA

Foreword

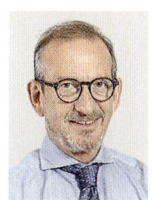

The evolution of endo-laparoscopic surgery together with information technology and digital transformation has dramatically changed even the innovative concept that minimal access surgery (MAS) brought in the early 1990'. This third edition of the "Recent Advances in Minimal Access Surgery" that will focus on Robotic and Innovative Surgery features the latest advance in MIS Innovation like robotic, operative endoscopic surgery and other surgical innovation by providing an updated to the Readers of the continuous evolution and development that we, as surgeons, are facing daily in our Operating Room. Ultimately, all these advances in surgery are focused on providing not only a better healthcare, but mainly an up-to-date and optimal outcome for our patients by reducing the trauma of the surgery and improving the results.

Prof Subash Khanna and all the Team from Indian Association for Gastrointestinal Endosurgeons (IAGES) have included in this textbook all the resources to make a compendium that will be useful for surgical residents, young surgeons and experts who want to master the latest advances in MAS.

Davide Lomanto
Professor of Surgery
Director of Minimally Invasive Surgery Centre
Yong Loo Lin School of Medicine
National University of Singapore

Preface

It is very heartening to share with readers that our earlier two editions of *Recent Advances in Minimal Access Surgery (RAMAS)* has been well accepted.

We all know change is the only constant. Change is imperative. Change is what leads to evolution. We, as surgeons have seen technology advance. Change is evident in almost everything we see in the OT—diathermy, OT table, scopes, insufflators, energy sources etc. Laparoscopy and endoscopic surgery brought a revolution in surgery. Suddenly surgeries were no longer painful. But as we know, laparoscopy has its share of limitations. This is where robotic surgery fills in. So basically with robotic surgery, we aspire to spread the benefits of minimal access surgery to all. Whether we like it or not, the day is not far when every OT will be mandatorily be equipped with a robot. With cheaper robots coming up, this is going to be faster than we anticipate. Anyone in denial of this fact will miss the bus to a better surgical experience and endless possibilities that one can explore with the improved manipulation and other technologies that come with the robot that strives for utmost precision. The evolution of surgery does not end in robotic surgery. Rather the surgical robot opens the floodgates of innovation. Things that we always thought of as part and parcel of surgery and accepted complications as our fate may no longer be so in near future. Let us take an example of anastomotic leak. Even the best of surgeons have borne the brunt of anastomotic leak. It usually happens if tissue compression is not ideal or vascularity is inadequate. Robotic staplers bring in the technology of perfecting tissue compression and the firefly technology tells us adequacy of vascularity at the anastomotic site, thus showing us a possibility of strictly leak free surgeries.

In the third edition of RAMAS, recognizing the importance of robot and disruptive technology that it brings along with the ability to eclipse the very way most of the surgeries are done today, we have decided to dedicate the 3rd edition of RAMAS to robotic surgery exclusively. In this edition, we have included a wide variety of articles encompassing the broad specialty of surgery along with its subspecialities, starting from the basics to very advanced procedures.

We have started our book with a chapter by me on current and upcoming robots to give an idea of the variety of robots that have stormed the market in various fields and their strengths. We have also tackled the very difficult and sensitive topic of robotic surgical training. There are chapters by Dr Raj Nagarkar et al., Dr Jignesh Gandhi et al., and Prof Shyamanta M Hazarika which tell us how robotic technology is shaping our future. We have included chapters written by the many other eminent robotic surgeons of the country—Robotic Esophageal Resections by Dr Kalyan Pandey, Colorectal Surgery by Dr Ahmed Pervez et al., TORS by Dr Kalpana Nagpal, Robotic Bariatric Surgery by Dr Arun Prasad and Robotic-assisted Revision Bariatric Surgery by Dr Sandeep Aggarwal, Robotic-assisted Liver Resection by Dr Gursev Sandlas, Pancreatic Surgery by Dr Amir Mushtaq Parray et al., and Robotic Hysterectomy by Dr Rooma Sinha. We have also included a chapter on PIPAC by Dr Hugo Teixeira Farinha in recognition to the fact that this minimally invasive palliative procedure may go a long way in improving the quality of life and prolong life.

I firmly believe that the way technology is progressing, we the doctors have no choice and we cannot progress further if we do not keep ourself updated with emerging technologies.

I am sure this book would give you a glimpse of some disrupted and Robotic technologies that are going to be a routine very soon.

Subhash Khanna

Contents

1. **Current and Upcoming Robots and Newer Technologies**............... 1
   Subhash Khanna

2. **Robotic Surgery: Training and Assessment** 20
   Matthew Boal, Nader Francis

3. **Development of Endoscopic Biliary Surgery Navigated by Artificial Intelligence** 37
   Yohei Kono, Masafumi Inomata, Seigo Kitano

4. **Machine Learning: Does it Prognosticate Colorectal Anastomotic Outcome?** 46
   Raj Nagarkar, Yasam Venkata Ramesh

5. **Precision Surgery in Rectal Resection Using Hyperspectral Imaging and Fluorescence Angiography** 59
   Jignesh Gandhi, Amay Banker

6. **Robotic Esophageal Resections: Improving Outcomes** 71
   Kalyan Pandey

7. **Perspectives on Robotic Colorectal Surgery in Today's World** 96
   Ahmed Pervez, Chelliah Selvasekar

8. **Robotic Transoral Surgery**.. 107
   Kalpana Nagpal

9. **PIPAC: Technique and Applications in Gastrointestinal Oncology** 120
   Hugo Teixeira Farinha, Amaniel Kefleyesus, Fabian Grass, Martin Hübner

10. **Robotic Bariatric Surgery** 138
    Arun Prasad

11. **Robot-assisted Liver Resection**... 145
    Gursev Sandlas

12. **Minimal Access and Robotic Surgery for Cystic Neoplasms of Pancreatic Body and Tail: Current Perspective**....................... 153
    Amir Mushtaq Parray, Ravindra Vats, Deep Goel

13. **Robotic-assisted Revision Bariatric Surgery** 169
    Arun Kumar, Vitish Singla, Prasanna Ramana, Sandeep Aggarwal

14. **Robotic Hysterectomy: How I do it?
    Sinha—Apollo Technique** 185
    Rooma Sinha, Bana Rupa, Mamtha Reddy

15. **Biomimetics and Artificial Intelligence: Pushing
    the Frontiers of Robotic Surgery** 193
    Shyamanta M Hazarika

Index *203*

CHAPTER 1
Current and Upcoming Robots and Newer Technologies

Subhash Khanna

■ INTRODUCTION

Ever since da Vinci received the Food and Drug Administration (FDA) approval in 2000, the world has witnessed the benefits of surgical robots. With the introduction of newer and affordable robots in the market, "robotic surgery" is the buzzword among surgeons today. The surgeries that were deemed difficult to do via laparoscopy for abdominal surgeries can now be done with relative ease with the robot. The robot also makes microdissection and suturing easier, due to which the robot now finds widespread acceptance by urologists, gynecologists, general surgeons, surgical oncologists, thoracic surgeons, and head and neck surgeons. Again, with the evolution of minimal access surgical techniques, there has been a steady advancement in the field of robotic endoscopy too. Robots have now been developed to make endoluminal surgery easier and take stereotactic bronchoscopic biopsies. *The world has seen a recent surge in the development of surgical robots and presently 96 surgical robots are being studied to be marketed for clinical use and of which 15 have received FDA approval.* So, the surgical robots can be broadly classified as:

- *Robotic minimal access surgical systems:*
  - Stereoscopic surgeon console systems
  - Open three-dimensional (3D) console systems
  - Single port (SP) systems [LESS (laparoendoscopic single-site) surgical systems]
- *Robotic endoscopy systems:*
  - Pure endoscopy/bronchoscopy systems
  - Endoscopic surgical systems
- Micro/nanobots

■ ROBOTS WITH STEREOSCOPIC SURGEON CONSOLE SYSTEMS

da Vinci® surgical system (Intuitive Surgical Inc., Mountain View, USA): This was the first commercially available surgical system that significantly impacted surgeons. This system has evolved over four generations and is still the leader in the robotic surgery market. The da Vinci SP model is a SP surgical system, in addition to Si, X, and Xi systems. Even though some of the important patents of Intuitive Surgical expired by 2019, they hold hundreds of more patents and are leaders in innovation and still ahead of their peers in the field of robotic surgery in various aspects such as wristed cameras, Iris technology, TilePro feature, dual console, Firefly technology, and choice of energy sources and staplers. The "Iris" technology uses data from diagnostic computed tomography (CT) imaging and creates a virtual 3D model. It aids in surgical planning which may lead to fewer complications, lesser confusion, and faster surgery. The "TilePro" feature allows for visualization of diagnostic images or 3D rendering of "Iris" images in a picture-on-picture fashion on the console screen for reference. The "Firefly" technology gives the robot to integrate fluorescence imaging using indocyanine green (ICG) or fluorescein dyes. The real-time near-infrared guidance enables the surgeon to more accurately identify the anatomy and even vascular perfusion, which in turn may lead to fewer iatrogenic injuries and fewer anastomotic leakages. Advanced bipolar energy devices are compatible with the da Vinci EndoWrist–SynchroSeal vessel sealer and vessel sealer extend. The sure form range of articulated staplers can move in a 120° cone of articulation giving tremendous maneuverability. They come in two lengths: 45 mm and 60 mm. The EndoWrist staplers 30 and 45 also allows for wristed articulation. With more than 6,700 installations worldwide, it is undoubtedly the market leader. Most of the evidence regarding robotic surgery that we have today is based on the da Vinci robot. The da Vinci SP system is the newest addition to the arsenal. It has shown quite promising results in urology, gynecology, and in cholecystectomy **(Fig. 1)**.[1-5]

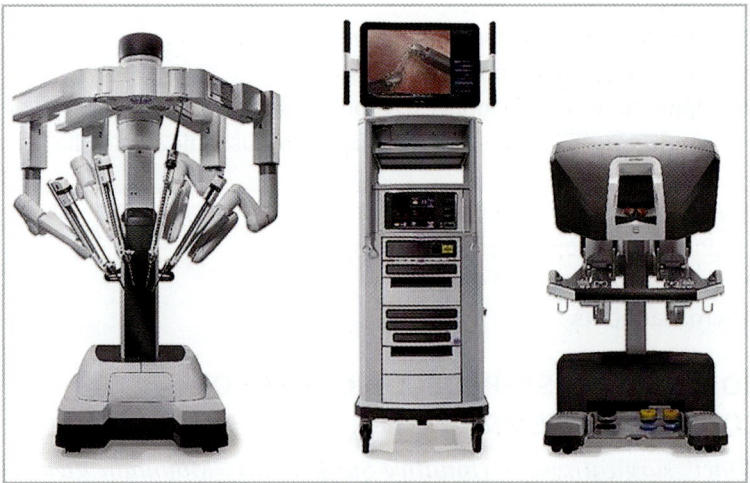

Fig. 1: Components of the da Vinci surgical system—patient cart, vision cart, and surgeon console.

Current and Upcoming Robots and Newer Technologies

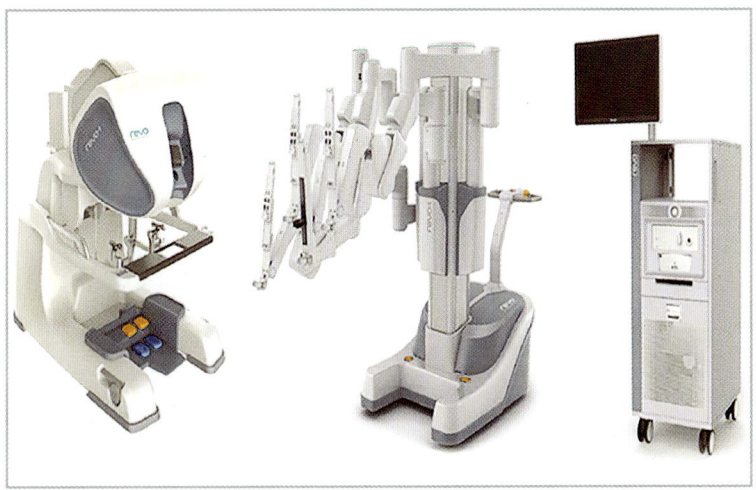

Fig. 2: Revo-i surgeon console and the four-arm robotic operation cart.

Revo-i® (Meerecompany Inc., Yongin, South Korea): The system obtained commercial approval from South Korea Ministry of Food and Drug Safety (MFDS) in August, 2017. The configuration of this surgical robot is similar to the da Vinci surgical system with an immersive display and robotic arms. It consists of a surgeon console, a four-arm robotic operation cart, a 3D high-definition (HD) vision cart, and reusable instrument. It differs from the da Vinci surgical system with regard to energy sources—currently it has only monopolar and bipolar energy delivery systems. It also lacks staplers and other advanced features that the da Vinci system offers. Revo-i surgical system has successfully demonstrated that it can safely carry out robotic-assisted radical prostatectomy (RARP), cholecystectomy, and can even carry out robotic reconstruction of pancreaticoduodenectomy. There are plans to launch the next model of Revo-i. Fairly complex surgeries have been found to be feasible on this platform including partial nephrectomy, central pancreatectomy, and pancreaticoduodenectomy **(Fig. 2)**.[6-8]

Hinotori surgical robotic system: This system was jointly developed by Kawasaki Heavy Industries and Sysmex, a medical company. It provides 3D HD vision on the stereoscopic viewer at the surgeon console just like the da Vinci platform. It is currently approved for use only in Japan. It consists of three components: the surgeon cockpit, the operation unit, and the vision unit. The robotic arms boast of 8 degrees of freedom **(Fig. 3)**.

■ OPEN CONSOLE SYSTEMS

Versius® (Cambridge Medical Robotics, Cambridgeshire, UK): It has the capability to allow robotic minimally invasive operations for a wide number of surgical procedures including gynecological, urological, head and neck,

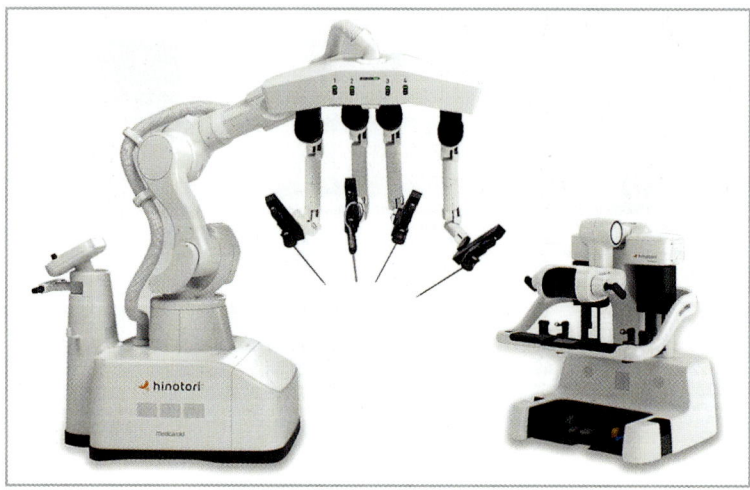

Fig. 3: Hinotori robotic system.

and colorectal surgical procedures.[9-15] It is a lightweight, multi-arm system, each with its own base in contrast to the da Vinci platform, which has arms attached to a single cart. It is an open console 3D HD system. The advantage of this system is that it has smaller arms requiring less space which can be moved around the operation tables (OTs), in contrast to the da Vinci platform which consumes considerable OT space. Up to four robotic arm ports can be used in addition to the camera port. Each arm is built like a human one, with three joints corresponding to the shoulder, the elbow, and the wrist. One of the main advantages with the system is that the robotic arms can be configured around the patient table in such a way that it accommodates a surgeon to operate laparoscopically, making way for hybrid robotic–laparoscopic surgery, which may be required in special clinical scenarios. The elbows of the robotic arms can be moved without changing the position of the instruments inside the abdomen, and can make some space for another surgeon to stand and assist at the bedside. It also boasts of motion scaling and haptic force feedback to the operator. One of the unique features of this system is the ability of the surgeon to stand at the console and operate if he desires so. The robotic arms use reusable instruments, which can be used up to 12 times. All the surgeries are stored in the cloud and the surgeons can review the previous surgeries, which may aid in learning and reduction in errors **(Fig. 4)**.

Hugo® RAS system (Medtronic, Minneapolis, MN, USA): It is a multi-arm, open console, 3D HD system like the Versius robotic platform. One of the strong points of this system is that it is compatible with the Covidien energy devices and staplers, which will be available in the future. Up to four robotic arms, including the endoscope can be connected for surgery. The life of each instrument varies for different instruments. It received CE mark approval

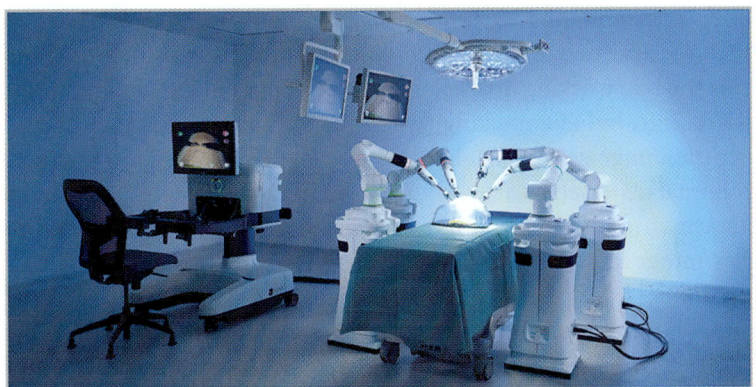

Fig. 4: The Versius robotic system has a surgeon console and four robotic arms in addition to the visualization arm.

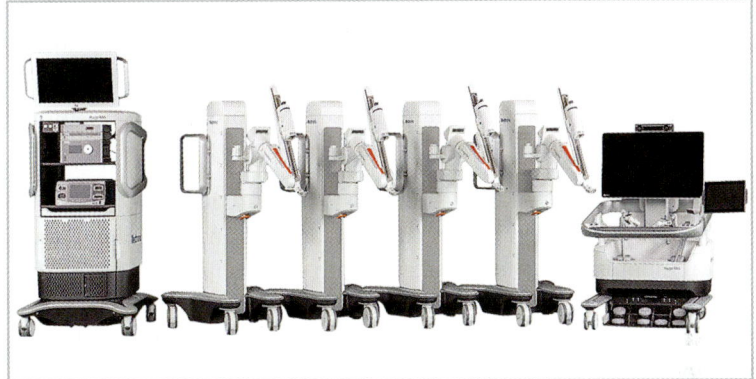

Fig. 5: Components of the Hugo RAS (robotic-assisted surgery) system–Hugo tower (central processing unit for the robotic system), arm carts, and surgeon console.

in October, 2021 authorizing the sale of the system in Europe for urologic and gynecologic procedures. It has also garnered FDA investigational device exemption (IDE) for clinical trials in the USA. It has shown feasibility in the performance of urological procedures. It has the ability to incorporate virtual reality/augmented reality via Microsoft HoloLens and includes a cloud-based surgical video capture option in Touch Surgery™ Enterprise with dedicated software modules to support robotics program optimization, and training options. Recent studies have shown that robotic-assisted prostatectomy on Hugo RAS (robotic-assisted surgery) system is safe and feasible **(Fig. 5)**.[16,17]

Senhance® (Asensus Surgical, formerly TransEnterix): Rather than a proper robotic platform, it can be addressed to as an advanced laparoscopic system given the limited choice of wristed instruments. Originally, FDA approved for gynecological surgeries, later FDA approval was acquired for general surgical procedures such as cholecystectomies, inguinal hernia repairs, and colorectal surgeries. The Senhance® system consists of a console that contains a screen, a keyboard, and two laparoscopic-type handles from which the surgeon controls the two working arms. Some of the unique features that this system offers are: infrared eye tracking (when the surgeon's head approaches the screen, the image zooms in), haptic force feedback, reusable instruments, and minimal disposables. It also has its own ultrasonic dissectors. It has three robotic arms in addition to the 3D camera. The controllers are like laparoscopy handles rather than joysticks. The working instruments are introduced into the abdominal cavity using commercially available laparoscopic trocars, and instruments can be resterilized for reuse. Some of the disadvantages of the current version of the Senhance® platform include the lack of articulating robotic instrumentation, a relatively limited variety of instruments that does not include stapling devices, and large arm booms connected to a separate console that consume considerable space both in the operating room and for storage. Again, sometimes haptic feedback is a disadvantage in situations where we need to retract a heavy organ for dissection. There is restriction of movement and makes dissection difficult. Even without wristed instruments, there is a fairly good evidence regarding use in various surgeries—urological, gynecological, colorectal, hernia, surgery, etc. **(Fig. 6)**.[18-23]

Micro Hand S: This surgical system has been indigenously developed by China. It has an open 3D surgeon console rather than an immersive display. The action mapping feature is available with three options: 1:3, 1:6, and 1:10. This means that moving 3, 6, or 10 cm at the surgeon console will translate to 1 cm movement of the operating arms. There is no limitation of the number of times the robotic instrument can be used. An ultrasonic scalpel can also be used with the robot. It has been touted as an affordable robot with less recurrent costs **(Fig. 7)**.

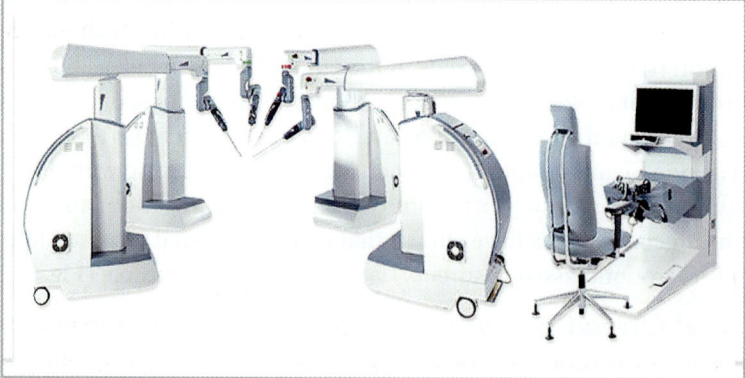

Fig. 6: The console is composed of a three-dimensional (3D) high-definition monitor, requiring specialized 3D glasses, an eye tracking camera, two master laparoscopic controllers, and a control pedal for instrument energy activation.

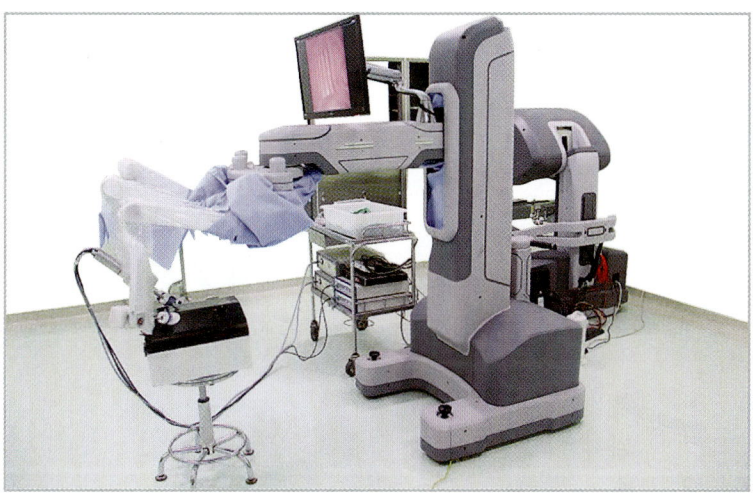

Fig. 7: The Micro Hand S surgical system.

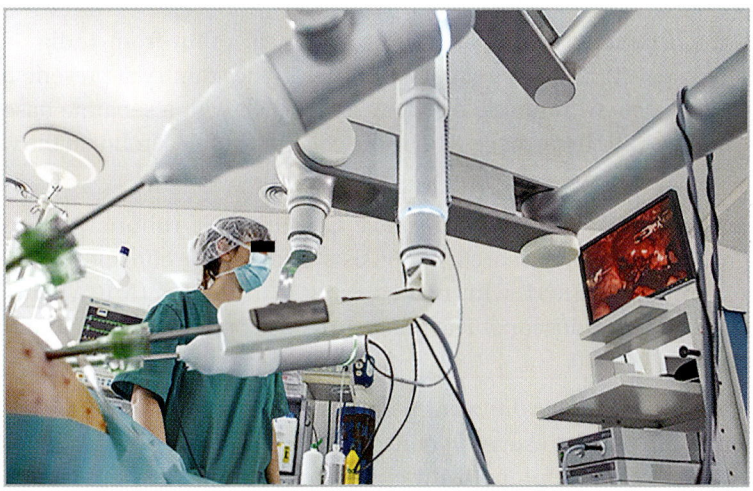

Fig. 8: Bitrack system.

Bitrack system (Rob Surgical Systems S.L., Barcelona, Spain): The prototype for this robotic system was finished in early 2015 and then moved into the clinical validation phase to gain approval for the European and US markets. It consists of a single cart with three robotic arms and an open-format surgeon console. The instruments are wristed with 7 degrees of freedom. Open-source ports allow both robotic and traditional lap instruments to operate simultaneously. Haptic feedback is available with this system. It has an open console with 3D HD screen. Robotic arms are mounted on a flexible floating fulcrum that proposes to enhance accessibility and access of the surgical cart around various patient positions. CE/FDA approvals are being processed **(Fig. 8)**.

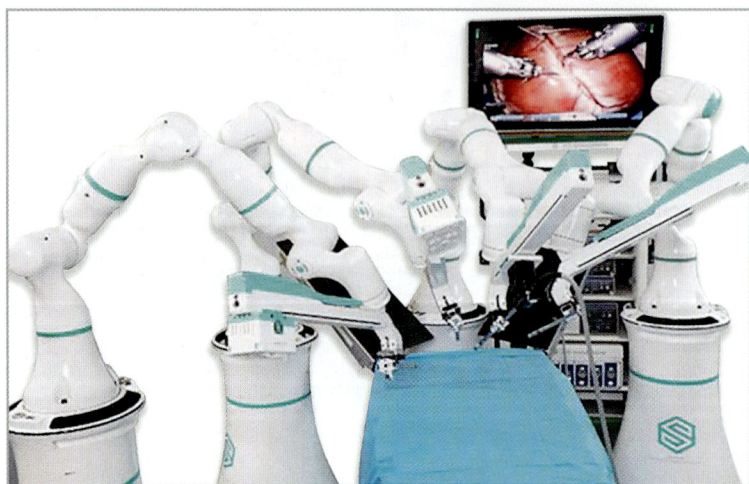

Fig. 9: The SSI Mantra robot components.

Mantra (SS innovations): It is the first surgical robot from India and is launched in 2022 and have two installations in the country at present. It has an open console with multiple robotic arms, each with a separate base like Hugo and Versius. It is expected to be the cheapest surgical robot in the world **(Fig. 9)**.

Microsurge (DLR, German Aerospace Centre): This robotic platform is designed mainly for research. It consists of a master console with three surgical robots (MIRO), with two carrying instruments (MICA) and one holding a stereo endoscope. The Microsurge was presented to the public for the first time in 2010.

Avatera surgical system (avateramedical GmbH, Germany): It is a robotic platform with an open surgeon console. It has four robotic arms including the endoscope. The unique feature is that they were able to decrease the diameter of the instruments to 5 mm. It received encumbrance certificate approval for the components of the surgical robotic system developed with Leibnitz University in 2019. It is undergoing further improvements.

Ottava: The Johnson & Johnson Ottava System is developed together with the company Verb Surgical (Santa Clara), founded in 2015.[16] It promises more flexibility and control than systems available today for soft tissue surgery. The new Ottava system has six arms that will be integrated into the operating table to provide greater control and flexibility in surgery. It was unveiled toward the end of 2020 and they are expected to start clinical trials from 2024.

Dexter (Distalmotion, Switzerland): This robotic surgical system is unique in the sense that it allows for quick undocking, and lets the sterile surgeon use laparoscopic instruments as and when required. Many a time the surgeon would like to use energy sources such as vessel sealers and ultrasonic scalpels which are not available with the newer robotic systems or would like to clip vessels in critical areas himself. In such a scenario, switching between laparoscopic and robotic platform helps, given that most of the surgeons have a good laparoscopy experience and may feel confident of some steps laparoscopically. It consists of two robotic arms whose range of motion is same as that of the other robotic systems. The conventional laparoscopic systems can be used with it.

■ LAPAROENDOSCOPIC SINGLE-SITE SURGICAL SYSTEMS

The Flex® Robotic System (Medrobotics®, Raynham, USA): It received United States Food and Drug Administration (US FDA) approval in July, 2015 for transoral and transrectal surgery. It provides the surgeon with SP access for operating on anatomical locations which are hard to reach via conventional instruments. In 2018, it also obtained FDA approval for obstetric/gynecologic applications. For transrectal surgery, it can reach up to distal sigmoid colon. It is a flexible camera-driven system with articulation with adjacent individual segments that can follow a nonlinear path just like a snake. The scope can be placed at a semirigid position to facilitate stabilization during surgery. It has channels on the side which can accommodate instruments such as a pair of scissors, needle driver, grasper, and dissector. Precise instrumentation with 3D vision is feasible in this platform. The surgeon sits or stands by the side of the patient with the 3D monitor in front and maneuvers the instruments. It does away with a bulky surgeon console. It can be equated with laparoscopy being done with semirigid instruments **(Fig. 10)**.

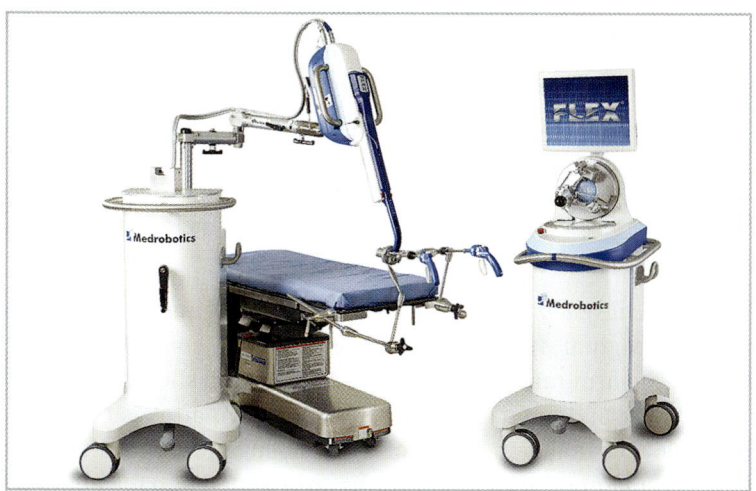

Fig. 10: The Flex robotic system.

10 Current and Upcoming Robots and Newer Technologies

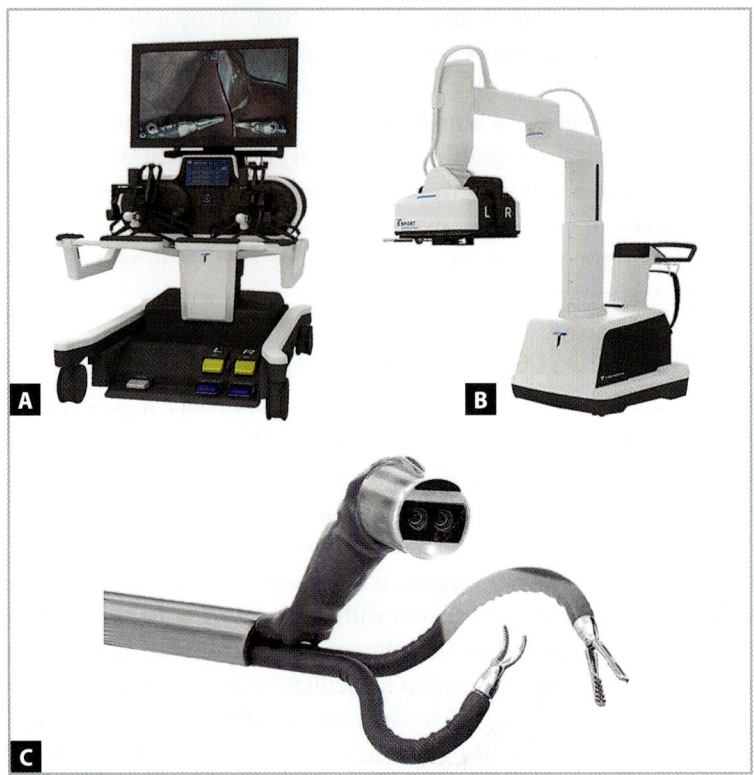

Figs. 11A to C: Titan SPORT. (A) Viewing console; (B) Surgical robot; (C) Flexible telescope with flexible robotic arms.

SPORT/Enos (Titan Medical, Toronto, Canada): SPORT abbreviates to SP orifice robotic technology. As the name suggests, it is an SP system. It has a stereoscopic viewing console with 3D HD vision with a flexible telescope and two flexible instruments. The two arms are inserted together but get separated once the surgeon starts dissection. All the components—multi-articulating instruments and integrated articulating 3D camera with lighting are passed through a single 25 mm incision. In a preclinical study performed on pigs and human cadaver, some of the abdominal procedures could be successfully performed.[24] It is very much like the da Vinci SP robotic platform **(Figs. 11A to C)**.

Hominis surgical system by MEMIC: Specifically designed to enable surgery via the transvaginal approach. There is only one small incision at the umbilicus. The arm mimics the human arm, having shoulder, elbow, and wrist inside the abdomen. The mobility of the two arms is unmatched—both have 360° flexibility in all directions enabling the surgeon to reach the whole of the abdomen. The robotic arms are inserted into the abdomen via the pouch of Douglas. A needle is first inserted under direct vision from the

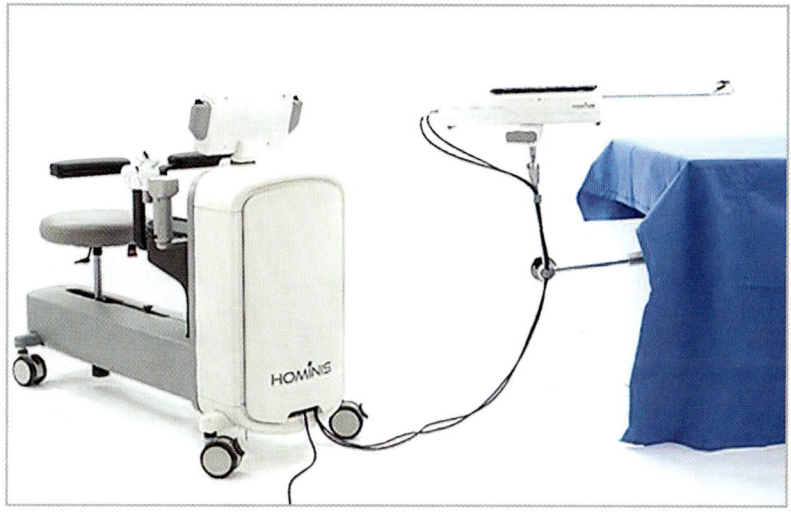

Fig. 12: The Hominis robotic platform.

camera inserted via the umbilicus. A blunt dilator is then inserted to create space for the arms cannula. The arms cannula is then positioned and robotic arms are inserted through the cannula. Both the robotic arms are controlled with the help of joysticks. Both the robotic arms can be used as graspers and both monopolar and bipolar cautery can be used for dissection. Ultrasonic dissectors and staplers are not available with this system. The surgeon console is open in this platform. It is US FDA approved for transvaginal hysterectomy for noncancerous conditions **(Fig. 12)**.

SurgiBot-SPIDER (single-port instrument delivery extended reach) (TransEnterix, Morrisville, NC): It could pass four instruments through a SP, with three robotic arms and 3D visualization. It underwent extensive preclinical testing but was rejected by the FDA in April, 2016. TransEnterix then sold the system to a Chinese medical device firm.

Vicarious surgical miniature robot (Vicarious Surgical, Waltham, US): It is mainly for hernia surgery. Current systems for surgery are disruptive—take a lot of space inside the operation theater and take long time to set up. It does away with the heavy equipment associated with the surgical robots currently available. They aim to launch the robot in 2023.

MIRA (miniaturized in vivo robotic assistant) Virtual Incision miniature robot (University of Nebraska): It is small, single-site surgery robotic platform. It may find utility for gallbladder and hernia surgery. This system consists of two arms with several miniature effectors such as graspers and monopolar cautery hook. The multiple joints on each arm make way for greater flexibility during surgical procedures. The endoscope and both the arms can be inserted

Current and Upcoming Robots and Newer Technologies

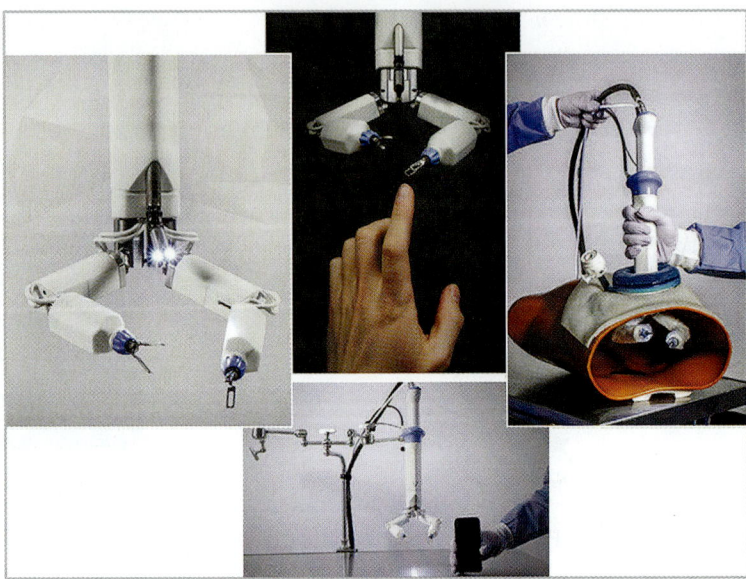

Fig. 13: MIRA (miniaturized in vivo robotic assistant) surgical robot platform.

via a single incision. The miniature robot can be easily positioned to access any quadrant of the abdomen **(Fig. 13)**.

ROBOTS CAPABLE OF ENDOLUMINAL SURGERY

The limitation with the current systems used for endoluminal surgery is that there is lack of triangulation and inadequate tissue retraction. The instrument and the camera move in the same axis and this creates an obstacle for proper dissection. These robots aim to overcome these limitations and make suturing, ligation, and retraction easy. This will hopefully make the endoluminal surgeries safer with lesser perforations and bleeding and less time consuming. They are still to come to the market, with most of them either in the preclinical stage or first human trials.

STRAS-iCUBE (iCUBE, Strasbourg, France): It is a flexible endoscopic system with instruments that can aid in intraluminal surgery. The STRAS (Single access and Transluminal Robotic Assistant for Surgeons) system features three modules: an endoscope module that drives four directions of deflection for the endoscope tip, instruments modules that enables the two ways of deflection for instruments, and translation and rotation modules (T/RMs) which rotate and translate the instruments within the channels of the main endoscope. It has a cable-driven system for instrumentation and camera movement. The modules allow for 10 degrees of freedom. This system is table mounted which saves space and enable quick set up. It is still in the preclinical stage.

EndoMaster EASE (Endoluminal Access Surgery Efficacy) System (Endomaster Pte Ltd., Singapore): It is one of the first endoscopic systems to be developed. In human trials are ongoing. It is meant for endoscopic removal of gastrointestinal (GI) tumors. The platform has a master console, a telesurgical work station and a robotic endoscope, with three instrument channels—one for insertion of conventional endoscopic instruments and the other two for robotic instruments—needle holder, cautery hook, and grasper, each having 9 degrees of freedom. In a prospective trial with five patients for gastric neoplasms, complete resection was achieved with this system.[25]

■ ENDOSCOPIC ROBOTS

Invendoscopy E210 system: It is a sterile-packed single-use colonoscopy system. It is controlled by invendoscope controller, which is detachable. It has one-handed controls for tip deflection, insufflation, suctioning, and image capture. The tip can deflect 180° in a very small radius. It features a special diagnostic mode, which magnifies the area viewed and can be well examined using the change of direction of the tip via hand controls. It has an instrument channel compatible with standard endoscopy instruments.

Monarch (Auris Surgical Robotics): It is basically a bronchoscope, operated with a joystick as in a gaming console. It can reach the most peripheral parts of the bronchial tree and perform biopsies. It combines virtual navigation to locate the tumors precisely. Once the robotic bronchoscope reaches the target lesion, it signals the operator to deploy needle for biopsy. Currently, a system that can ablate the target lesions is being developed and is expected to be available soon.

Ion (Intuitive Surgical Inc., Mountain View, USA): It is a robotic bronchoscopy platform much like the Monarch platform, specifically designed to take biopsies from peripheral lung nodules which are not amenable for biopsy with the conventional bronchoscopes. Such nodules are usually small and cannot be reliably targeted by an intervention radiologist. Again, there is an associated risk of pneumothorax on repeated attempts in such a situation. It has a thin 3.5 mm maneuverable scope, which can move 180°, is stable and flexible enough to reach peripheral airways. Prior to the procedure, the Plan Point software uses CT scan of the lungs to generate 3D images to create a preplanned path for bronchoscopic biopsy, which is loaded to the system. With Ion's vision probe, the physician gains real-time vision of the airway. It has the capability to take biopsies from even extraluminal masses.

Robotics for Specific Purpose

- *THINK Surgical's Tsolution One:* It is specifically designed for total knee arthroplasty (TKA) and is FDA cleared for the specific purpose. Other

systems used for this purpose are Velys robotic-assisted solution by Johnson and Johnson and Mako robot by Stryker.
- *Restoration Robotics' ARTAS:* It is specifically designed for hair transplant—chooses the best follicles for implant, cuts them out, and makes tiny incisions for the transplants.
- *Mazor Robotics' Renaissance:* It is specifically designed for spinal surgery. Prior to surgery, the software uses 3D scans to analyze the patients' anatomy. It finds areas of symmetry and helps the surgeon make decisions. The 3D syncing system maps the scans to the patient vertebra by vertebra. During surgery, a guidance unit positions the surgeon's instruments allowing for 1.5 mm accuracy. The latest Mazor X Stealth Edition integrates the Medtronic stealth navigation technology with the O-arm interoperable scanner in its robotic platform.
- *Medical Microinstruments' (MMI's) Symani robotic microsurgery system:* It is for intracavitary microsurgery and open microsurgical procedures. The system combines the benefits of tremor reduction and motion scaling (7–20x) with the world's smallest wristed instrumentation. The system's NanoWrist instruments are designed to overcome the challenges of free-flap reconstructions, replantations, congenital malformations, peripheral nerve repairs, and lymphatic surgery **(Fig. 14)**.
- *Sensei X robotic catheter system (Hansen Medical Inc., Mountain View, California):* It is primarily intended for use in cardiovascular procedures requiring the use of a catheter. The movement of each component is driven by traction wires via a remote joystick or buttons on the main console. Information from 3D mapping, intracardiac echocardiography (ICE), fluoroscopy, and electrocardiogram (ECG) recordings are integrated

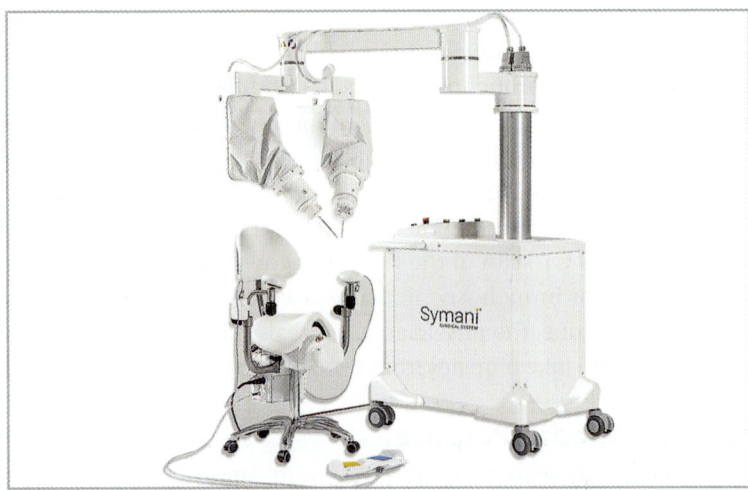

Fig. 14: Symani robotic microsurgery system.

with navigation system for accurate positioning and manipulation. Other similar systems for cardiovascular procedures are vascular catheter CorPath GRX, Aeon Phocus cardiac catheter, and Siemens Healthineers vascular robotics.
- *VIKY (Endocontrol Medical, La Tronche, France):* VIKY EP is a video endoscope positioner and VIKY UP is a motorized uterine manipulator. It provides direct control of the surgeon in the camera positioning. The manipulation is via multilingual voice activation or foot activation. It has the ability to memorize key positions. It frees an assistant from holding the camera and also lets the surgeon have a view of his choice without shaking of image. It is a light-weight robot, which is fixed to the operating table rail and adjustable during surgery.
- *The MrBot equipment:* It is used in conjunction with the magnetic resonance imaging (MRI) for interventions in the prostate gland. It is designed for transperineal needle insertion and performance of percutaneous interventions such as biopsy, thermal ablations, or brachytherapy.
- *Micromate robot (Interventional Systems, Austria):* It is a miniature robot that can guide image-guided interventions such as biopsy and may prove invaluable for oncology. It has received FDA 510(k) clearance for percutaneous procedures.
- *XACT ACE robotic system:* It functions similar to the Micromate robot. It is used for intervention radiology procedures. The system is used for trajectory planning and is intended to assist the physician in positioning of an instrument, such as a needle, where CT imaging is used for target trajectory planning and intraoperative tracking. It has also received FDA 510(k) clearance for percutaneous procedures.
- *The AcuBot and Revolving Needle Driver equipment:* It is developed for enhanced accuracy of nephrolithotomy.
- *Freehand collaborative robot*: It has the following components—the control box powers the robotic motion assembly. The headset allows the surgeon to select the direction of the scope movement. The indicator unit is in line with the surgeon's headset and placed above the monitor at the midpoint. It has motion sensors that detect the surgeon's head movement which in turn, moves the camera via activation of the foot pedals. Remote camera zoom is also feasible with this platform. It is lightweight and can easily be attached to the frame by the side of the operating table.
- *The LAP Mentor equipment (Simbionix):* Try surgeries on a virtual patient.
- *Axesse equipment:* For precise radiation therapy
- *Retraction Robot:* For SP systems, magnetic-based retraction
- *Scorpion-shaped endoscopic robot*: For natural orifice transluminal endoscopic surgery (NOTES) and LESS

- *VERB surgical (Google + Johnson and Johnson):* It is a digital surgery platform but not a robot. It is touted to be an open and flexible system that will allow the integration of open, laparoscopic, and robotic surgery with superior software and data analytics.
- *EndoAID (Olympus):* Detection of polyps via artificial intelligence (AI)
- *PowerSpiral enteroscope (Olympus):* It is a motorized endoscope which has the capacity to examine the whole of small intestine.

Capsule Endoscopy

They have a wide variety of clinical utility, starting from diagnostics like taking a biopsy to therapeutics. One such surgical robot has a nitinol clip, which is loaded at the topside of the capsule and was successfully able to clip iatrogenic bleed in the sigmoid colon. The capsule was guided by means of external magnetic guidance.[26] It is a significant development considering that it was able to do an autonomous task. This modality of therapeutics does away with the invasive procedures currently done for the same purpose and brings forward greater possibilities for other therapeutic interventions.

■ MICRO-ROBOTS (MICROBOTS)

These are basically robots smaller than 1 mm. Microbots are the next frontier in robotic technology. Till now we have seen tethered robots (robots having no autonomy and controlled entirely by the surgeon console). These are untethered systems that have a certain degree of autonomy and can take actions based on certain tissue characteristics. The microrobotic instruments must contain four key characteristics for successful development: contained propulsion, miniaturized functionality, accurate telemanipulation, and consistent visualization. These systems are still in the preclinical phase but will be available soon.

Microbots will find applications in eye surgery, within the vascular space, interstitial tissue, and GI tract. They may be either externally driven like a magnetic field or ultrasonographic energy, or they may be self-propulsive (internally-driven) via controlled chemical reactions. For a surgical microbot to be functional, it should be able to do what surgical instruments are capable of—dissecting, grasping, and ablation at a micro scale. One of the studies utilized a rapidly vibrating micropipette for dissection of neurons at a micro level.[27] Spring-driven microspikes, originally conceptualized for capsule endoscopes, can also be used for cutting. Grasping can be done with the help of chemical changes or thermal energy.[27,28] Ablative surgical maneuvers can be actuated via high energy projective robots that are directed into specific tissue types.[29]

■ CONCLUSION

Since the launch of da Vinci surgical system in 1999, it has enjoyed monopoly, thanks to the 649 US patents to its name. But many of the patents of the da Vinci system has expired since the end of 2016 like its remote controls, arm joints, and automatic adjustments on the positioning of endoscopes. Many more patents will expire in the next few years. With the surgical robotics market to grow to $24 billion by 2025, a lot of competitors have ventured into this space. The testimony of this fact is that 96 robots are ready to be marketed and 15 have already gained FDA approval. All these surgical robots have to be cheaper, better, or specialized for a certain task to claim market share from Intuitive Surgical. With specific needs for each of the specialty, specialized robots having features specific to that specialty have come up. It is to be seen if they stand up to the test of time.

Given that there are a lot of robotic platforms in the market today, it seems many more players will enter the market soon. In the war for dominance in this field, it seems that the robot having the most responsive arm will not win the race, rather the one who will integrate a range of technologies at the machine's disposal such as augmented/virtual reality, integration of clinical images and data, machine learning and automated tasks, advanced imaging techniques, and having wide range of energy devices at their disposal.

■ REFERENCES

1. Dobbs RW, Halgrimson WR, Madueke I, Vigneswaran HT, Wilson JO, Crivellaro S. Single-port robot-assisted laparoscopic radical prostatectomy: initial experience and technique with the da Vinci® SP platform. BJU Int. 2019;124(6):1022-7.
2. Moschovas MC, Bhat S, Sandri M, Rogers T, Onol F, Mazzone E, et al. Comparing the Approach to Radical Prostatectomy Using the Multiport da Vinci Xi and da Vinci SP Robots: A Propensity Score Analysis of Perioperative Outcomes. Eur Urol. 2021;79(3):393-404.
3. Kaouk J, Garisto J, Eltemamy M, Bertolo R. Step-by-step technique for single-port robot-assisted radical cystectomy and pelvic lymph nodes dissection using the da Vinci® SPTM surgical system. BJU Int. 2019. [Online ahead of print]
4. Heo JE, Kang SK, Koh DH, Na JC, Lee YS, Han WK, et al. Pure single-site robot-assisted pyeloplasty with the da Vinci SP surgical system: Initial experience. Investig Clin Urol. 2019;60(4):326-30.
5. Shin HJ, Yoo HK, Lee JH, Lee SR, Jeong K, Moon HS. Robotic single-port surgery using the da Vinci SP® surgical system for benign gynecologic disease: A preliminary report. Taiwan J Obstet Gynecol. 2020;59(2):243-7.
6. Kang I, Hwang HK, Lee WJ, Kang CM. First experience of pancreaticoduodenectomy using Revo-i in a patient with insulinoma. Ann Hepatobiliary Pancreat Surg. 2020;24(1):104-8.
7. Ku G, Kang I, Lee WJ, Kang CM. Revo-i assisted robotic central pancreatectomy. Ann Hepato-Biliary-Pancreat Surg. 2020;24(4):547-50.
8. Kim DK, Park DW, Rha KH. Robot-assisted Partial Nephrectomy with the REVO-I Robot Platform in Porcine Models. Eur Urol. 2016;69(3):541-2.

9. Puntambekar SP, Rajesh KN, Goel A, Hivre M, Bharambe S, Chitale M, et al. Colorectal cancer surgery: by Cambridge Medical Robotics Versius Surgical Robot System-a single-institution study. Our experience. J Robot Surg. 2022;16(3):587-96.
10. Atallah S, Parra-Davila E, Melani AGF. Assessment of the Versius surgical robotic system for dual-field synchronous transanal total mesorectal excision (taTME) in a preclinical model: will tomorrow's surgical robots promise newfound options? Tech Coloproctol. 2019;23(5):471-7.
11. Thomas BC, Slack M, Hussain M, Barber N, Pradhan A, Dinneen E, et al. Preclinical Evaluation of the Versius Surgical System, a New Robot-assisted Surgical Device for Use in Minimal Access Renal and Prostate Surgery. Eur Urol Focus. 2021;7(2):444-52.
12. Faulkner J, Arora A, Swords C, Cook E, Rajangam A, Jeannon JP. Pre-clinical evaluation of a novel robotic system for transoral robotic surgery. Clin Otolaryngol. 2021;46(4):869-74.
13. Kelkar DS, Kurlekar U, Stevens L, Wagholikar GD, Slack M. An Early Prospective Clinical Study to Evaluate the Safety and Performance of the Versius Surgical System in Robot-Assisted Cholecystectomy. Ann Surg. 2022. [Online ahead of print]
14. Kelkar D, Borse MA, Godbole GP, Kurlekar U, Slack M. Interim safety analysis of the first-in-human clinical trial of the Versius surgical system, a new robot-assisted device for use in minimal access surgery. Surg Endosc. 2021;35(9):5193-202.
15. Morton J, Hardwick RH, Tilney HS, Gudgeon AM, Jah A, Stevens L, et al. Preclinical evaluation of the versius surgical system, a new robot-assisted surgical device for use in minimal access general and colorectal procedures. Surg Endosc. 2021;35(5):2169-77.
16. Bravi CA, Paciotti M, Sarchi L, Mottaran A, Nocera L, Farinha R, et al. Robot-assisted Radical Prostatectomy with the Novel Hugo Robotic System: Initial Experience and Optimal Surgical Set-up at a Tertiary Referral Robotic Center. Eur Urol. 2022;82(2):233-7.
17. Ragavan N, Bharathkumar S, Chirravur P, Sankaran S, Mottrie A. Evaluation of Hugo RAS System in Major Urologic Surgery: Our Initial Experience. J Endourol. 2022;36(8):1029-35.
18. Samalavicius NE, Janusonis V, Siaulys R, Jasėnas M, Deduchovas O, Venckus R, et al. Robotic surgery using Senhance® robotic platform: single center experience with first 100 cases. J Robot Surg. 2020;14(2):371-6.
19. Montlouis-Calixte J, Ripamonti B, Barabino G, Corsini T, Chauleur C. Senhance 3-mm robot-assisted surgery: experience on first 14 patients in France. J Robot Surg. 2019;13(5):643-7.
20. Schmitz R, Willeke F, Barr J, Scheidt M, Saelzer H, Darwich I, et al. Robotic Inguinal Hernia Repair (TAPP) First Experience with the New Senhance Robotic System. Surg Technol Int. 2019;34:243-9.
21. Kaštelan Ž, Knežević N, Hudolin T, Kuliš T, Penezić L, Goluža E, et al. Extraperitoneal radical prostatectomy with the Senhance Surgical System robotic platform. Croat Med J. 2019;60(6):556-9.
22. Darwich I, Stephan D, Klöckner-Lang M, Scheidt M, Friedberg R, Willeke F. A roadmap for robotic-assisted sigmoid resection in diverticular disease using a Senhance™ Surgical Robotic System: results and technical aspects. J Robot Surg. 2020;14(2):297-304.

23. Kastelan Z, Hudolin T, Kulis T, Knezevic N, Penezic L, Maric M, et al. Upper urinary tract surgery and radical prostatectomy with Senhance® robotic system: Single center experience-First 100 cases. Int J Med Robot. 2021;17(4):e2269.
24. Seeliger B, Diana M, Ruurda JP, Konstantinidis KM, Marescaux J, Swanström LL. Enabling single-site laparoscopy: the SPORT platform. Surg Endosc. 2019;33(11):3696-703.
25. Phee SJ, Reddy N, Chiu PWY, Rebala P, Rao GV, Wang Z, et al. Robot-assisted endoscopic submucosal dissection is effective in treating patients with early-stage gastric neoplasia. Clin Gastroenterol Hepatol. 2012;10(10):1117-21.
26. Valdastri P, Quaglia C, Susilo E, Menciassi A, Dario P, Ho CN, et al. Wireless therapeutic endoscopic capsule: in vivo experiment. Endoscopy. 2008;40(12):979-82.
27. Kirson ED, Yaari Y. A novel technique for micro-dissection of neuronal processes. J Neurosci Methods. 2000;98(2):119-22.
28. Singh AV, Sitti M. Targeted Drug Delivery and Imaging Using Mobile Milli/Microrobots: A Promising Future Towards Theranostic Pharmaceutical Design. Curr Pharm Des. 2016;22(11):1418-28.
29. Kagan D, Benchimol MJ, Claussen JC, Chuluun-Erdene E, Esener S, Wang J. Acoustic droplet vaporization and propulsion of perfluorocarbon-loaded microbullets for targeted tissue penetration and deformation. Angew Chem Int Ed Engl. 2012;51(30):7519-22.

CHAPTER 2

Robotic Surgery: Training and Assessment

Matthew Boal, Nader Francis

■ INTRODUCTION

Over the past three decades, there has been a rapid uptake of minimally invasive surgery (MIS), laparoscopic and robotic techniques, across different specialties. Robotic surgery is a well-established modality; since the introduction of da Vinci robotic surgical system in 2000 and has since been used in more than 8.5 million procedures, 1.25 million of which were in 2020.[1] Initially, it was developed and introduced to cardiac surgery, subsequently it was adopted in many subspecialties and nowadays urology is the specialty to truly adopt it as minimally invasive technique.[2]

Perceived advantages of robotic surgery include ergonomics for the surgeon, improved depth of field vision with 3D visualization of the operative field, increased stabilization, and dexterity with instruments.[3]

There is evidence showing improved ergonomics with robotics versus laparoscopic and open, predominantly by improving posture[4] as well as arm and shoulder positions. One study using validated tools showed better scores for postural analysis in robotics versus laparoscopy.[5] Surgeons reported pain in pelvic surgery with 50% after laparotomy, 56% in laparoscopy, and 23% after robotics.[6] In a dry study, ergonomics and performance improved, as well as reduced mental stress/cognitive load in surgical novices when comparing robotic to laparoscopic tasks.[7]

When comparing 2D versus 3D in MIS, some early small studies showed reduced error rates[8] including skills-based error by 93%.[9] The European Association of Endoscopic Surgery (EAES) suggested that 3D vision reduces operative times, particularly in cases with laparoscopic suturing, as well as reduced errors in dry lab simulation.[10] The evidence in experimental labs is in favor of robotics performing better than standard laparoscopy when performing complex tasks,[4] usually suturing and knot tying tasks.

Dexterity is the ability to perform a difficult action quickly or skillfully with the hands.[11] Although there is no clinical data on the degrees of freedom to perform a task well, laparoscopy has four degrees of freedom and is backed up with clinical data as to its effectiveness. A robotic arm has an outer and inner joint so giving it six degrees of freedom, mimicking a human hand

and arm articulation. A seventh degree of freedom in a robotic arm can be considered with jaw movement. Intuitive's da Vinci system was the first laparoscopic robotic system to incorporate six degrees of freedom in 2000.[2] A study showed that the presence of wristed instrumentation, tremor abolition, and motion scaling by robotic systems enhance dexterity by nearly 50% as compared to laparoscopic surgery.[9] This may account for data suggesting a reduced learning curve for robotic technical skills when compared to laparoscopy.[12,13]

Perceived disadvantages mostly relate to lack of haptic feedback, potentially increasing the risk of iatrogenic injury, although, several new models have incorporated automated haptic feedback.[14] Cost-effectiveness is a concern in robotic surgery, many American studies comparing the cost of robotic-assisted to laparoscopic surgery showed it is more expensive, with longer operating times.[2]

It is hypothesized with the enhancement of technology that this will lead to reduced error, improved patient outcome through reduced complications and length of stay, along with increased annual throughput with improved portability of newer systems; this will offset the cost of training and purchase.[2]

As we progress in healthcare, we must expect to have increased expenditure in pharmaceuticals and medical devices, in order to remain at the forefront of surgical technology whilst maintaining competency, given the increasing public and professional scrutiny of surgical performance and patient safety.

IMPORTANCE OF TRAINING AND VALIDATED CURRICULA IN ROBOTIC SURGERY

Error in Surgery and Robotics

With an increasing use of robotic systems across different specialties, there is an ongoing call for standardization of training, assessment, testing and credentialing.[15] A study from the USA reported 10,624 adverse events relating to robotic procedures between 2000 and 2013.[16] Experts raised concerns over surgical curricula being random and insufficient to ensure patient safety,[17] leading to the development of EAU Robotic Urology Section Curriculum (ERUS). In addition, an independent review by the Emergency Care Research Institute (ECRI) on health technology hazards identified a lack of robotic surgical training as one of the top 10 risks to patients.[18,19] Comparisons are frequently made between the aviation industry and surgery in terms of adverse event analysis and nontechnical skills. The aviation industry, however, has mandatory, recurrent, reassessment, and requalification throughout the career pathway and an internationally agreed standard for training, which robotic surgery does not.[19,20]

Describing the "Swiss Cheese Effect" Reason in 2000 identified errors in health care with a systems-based approach rather than individual blame. Reason highlighted four main areas to reduce human error and improve patient safety.[19,21]
1. Policy writing and training
2. Standardization and simplification
3. Automation
4. Improvement of devices and architecture.

In robotic surgery, these processes described earlier are being addressed but still need more research and development.

Work is needed still to develop and validate curricula to globally standardize training and certification of robotic surgery within each specialty,[22] however, accepting that there will geographical and financial differences in the ability to provide certain elements, e.g., cadavers, dual console training. Considering these limitations, we must explore alternative ways to improve training and accessibility for all.

Robotic Training Curricula

A proposed framework for development of curricula in any branch of medicine for learning a technical skill, five steps are recommended:[23]
1. Knowledge-based learning
2. Deconstruction of the procedures into component tasks
3. Training in a skills laboratory environment
4. Demonstration of transfer of skills to the real environment
5. Assessment of competency to enable granting of privileges for independent practice.

Initial curricula introduced include fundamentals of robotic surgery (FRS), fundamentals skills of robotic surgery (FSRS) and urology have introduced the first validated specialty curriculum, EAU Robotic Urology Section Curriculum (ERUS),[22,24] from which British Association of Urological Surgeons (BAUS) based their curriculum.[25] Other curricula exist now within specialties including thoracics,[26] gynecology[27] and general surgery, but none have been standardized.

In 2020, the Orsi Consensus Meeting on European Robotic Training (OCERT)[28], had 36 international experts identify and agree on 23 key statements, based on three themes:
- Training Standardization pathways
- Validation metrics i.e. objective assessment
- Implementation prerequisites and certification.

Other key aspects included accreditation should be awarded by the relevant professional societies and/or universities.

Fundamentals of Robotic Surgery and FSRS are both simulation-based. FRS has four modules spanning from pre- to postoperative, focusing on all aspects including didactic teaching, psychomotor skills, team training, and communication skills with the aim to teach generic robotic skills and cognitive modules to surgeons from any specialty. It has been validated in a recent RCT showing better performance of those trained following FRS compared to controls.[29] It also boasts a free app, taking the student through Intuitive systems training and with a validated, expert created, cognitive test at the end. This allows for one of the steps to be achieved set out by OCERT which there was 100% consensus on that "pre-course e-learning evaluation be completed to a sufficient standard (benchmarked) before attending a basic robotic skills training course". It should be noted that the FRS and e-learning is only relevant to da Vinci robotic systems, as such, similar methods will have to developed and evaluated for other robotic systems. FSRS is validated and assessed by the Robotic Skills Assessment Score tool. ERUS follows a more comprehensive model of didactic online teaching, simulation with dry, wet and live lab training including procedure-specific assessment. The next stage is a fellowship including observation, bedside assisting, dual console mentoring until independent in a procedure and certification with a theoretical and practical examination.[24,25] ERUS, similarly to FSRS, concludes simulation training with summative assessments, using GEARS and a theoretical examination.[25] There are some concerns, however, over the generalizability of ERUS across lower volume centers. The program was piloted in a higher volume center which is potentially why the desired training goals were achieved.[28]

Robotic procedure-specific sign off recommendations by BAUS differ per procedure but broadly focus on the total number of logbook cases and certain objective outcome measures, e.g., operative time, estimated blood loss, positive resection margins, and complication rate.[25] This misses an additional opportunity to analyze intraoperative skill and errors, rather, looking at patient outcomes as an indicator of competency.

Learning Curve

The learning or proficiency gain curve is defined in surgery as the start point, the slope and then the plateau of that individual,[29] i.e., the number of procedures a surgeon needs to perform to reach a plateau in relation to specified outcomes such as operating time, conversion rates, complication and mortality.[30]

When implementing a technique or a new intervention, the learning curve must be considered and ways to shorten it effectively should be taken into account. The move to proficiency-based training, rather than traditional time-based curricula is based upon clearly defined training endpoints for the trainee. It allows an opportunity for performance review and setting new targets as they progress along the learning curve. Feedback on performance is provided and leads to enhanced skill acquisition.[31]

The definition of competency is usually based on a summative assessment and case numbers usually quoted at around 15–25 per case type. However, total case number alone is a crude tool to assess competence. A meta-analysis showed the mean number of procedures to become "expert" across various specialties was 39.[20,32] The environment in which learning is taking place must also be considered. An "institutional" learning curve was demonstrated in one study showing that case numbers to become competent were 74 when a new robotic service was set up, reducing to 25–30 once it was well established.[20,33] This shortened learning curve could be due to improved team training and supervisor knowledge. Additionally, the concept of interspecialty proctors could be used to enhance learning of generic robotic skills.[20]

One theme identified in the learning curve by ERUS, while developing the curriculum was identifying the needs of the trainees who often have exposure to minimally invasive surgery. However, there seems to be no difference in the learning curve for robotic skills in those who are laparoscopically trained with those who perform mostly open.[29,34] One study found that there was no negative impact on the learning curve of a novice with no previous laparoscopic or even open urological experience.[35]

ERUS curriculum discusses that case load alone is not enough to assess proficiency in robotic skills and procedures. The ERUS curriculum basic layout is seen in **Figure 1**.

E-Learning

There is growing evidence supporting the effectiveness of e-learning on clinician performance and patient outcomes.[36] It can enhance access to learning including standardization and accessibility globally. It will undoubtedly help with initial knowledge acquisition and can incorporate non-technical skills key to robotic, or any, surgery.

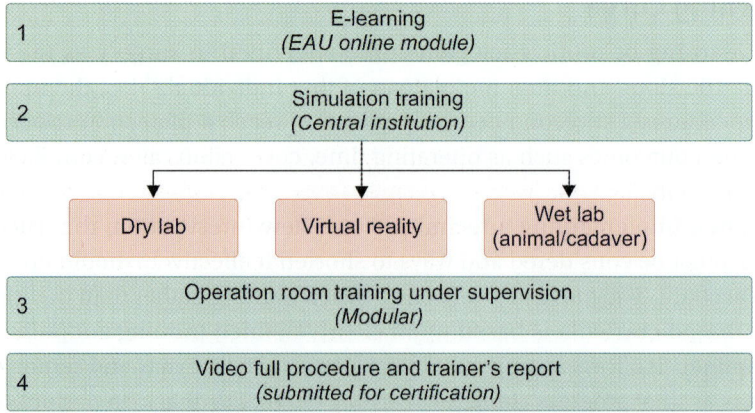

Fig. 1: ERUS proposed curriculum.[17]

E-learning can provide effective task demonstration; comprehensive, standardized instruction and demonstration to understand and acquire skills or procedures.[37] Normally task demonstration is unstructured through verbal feedback intraoperatively, however, this misses an opportunity preoperatively to enhance learning through video-based tutorials.

Simulation-based Training

Training in robotics is difficult due to the time constraints of working hours, availability, and financial constraints.[38] Simulation is, therefore, a key element to shorten the learning curve before and during observership/mentorship programs.[39] Validated virtual reality simulation platforms exist including Mimic dV-trainer, ProMIS, Sim Surgery Educational Platform (SEM) and Intuitive Systems showing construct, face and content validity[38] with level 2 and 3 evidence,[40] while the Robotic Surgical Simulator system demonstrates face and content validity.[17] There is a lack of evidence for the predictive validity of most VR simulators,[41] however, a meta-analysis in 2021 demonstrated skill and predictive validity of da Vinci Skills Simulator (dvS) and Mimic dV-Trainer.[42] Additionally, one study in laparoscopy showed improved operative performance in laparoscopic cholecystectomy after VR simulation.[43]

Simulation training in the dry and wet lab allows progression through the learning curve without compromise to patient safety and is shown to be transferable to clinical practice.[44] Although in some regions geographically there may be cost and ethical issues for wet lab use (cadaver or animal),[45] however, VR and dry lab simulation are both validated and widely available tools for training and assessment. Additionally, simulation-based training is proven to be an invaluable teaching method for non-technical skills outside of robotics in medical and aviation training. Within postgraduate medicine, it is a useful tool for clinical and performance based formative assessment[46] containing feedback sessions which are key to bridgeing knowledge gaps.

Simulation with animal, fresh frozen or Thiel embalmed cadavers are considered the highest fidelity. Live animal replicates intraoperative physiological conditions and human cadavers represent accurate anatomy.

The next step in for high fidelity, simulation training is 3D printing, with existing validated and cost-effective compared to animal and cadaver, mostly within urology.[40] Novel 3D printed models using hydrogel casting methods have created a surgical rehearsal platform and a reasonable alternative to cadaver or animal tissues. Results have shown similar mechanical and functional properties of hydrogel polyvinyl alcohol (PVA) kidneys compared to those of a live kidney.[47] In addition, objective metrics can be simulated for assessment including blood loss, tissue tension through tensiometers and tumor resection margins through UV light examination. This novel non-biohazardous simulation excludes ethical/religious issues, infection and safety risks, as well as reducing financial costs.[48]

PROCTORING/PRECEPTORING, MENTORING, FELLOWSHIPS AND ASSESSMENT

Proctoring/preceptoring is the observation of a surgeon by a trainer during the initial phase of the proficiency gain curve, i.e., a trainee observed by someone experienced, in order to assess their knowledge and skills of the new procedure/technique. In robotics, this is the key to accreditation of surgeons but also of institutions who are proctoring, to ensure safe acquisition of skills before going on to independent practice.[49]

Mentoring is training when an experienced surgeon in a technique supervises with the intention to guide acquisition of a new skill, e.g., robotics, in the steep part of the proficiency gain curve, therefore, ideally be independent of performance review. Mentoring can point out strengths and help overcome difficulties experienced by the trainee through "tips and tricks".[49]

In the UK, the National Institute for Health and Care Excellence (NICE) in 2006 suggested laparoscopic surgery be offered to all appropriate colorectal cancer patients. However, it had to be waived initially as it was recognized only a minority of surgeons could provide training. This resulted in the National Training Programme for Laparoscopic Colorectal Surgery (LAPCO) being set up by the Department of Health, England.[20,50] The LAPCO scheme thought that 20 cases would be enough to become competent but recognized that there would be variation. This competency-based training program involved a sign off process by which surgeons in training had to submit two videos of complete, unedited, laparoscopic colorectal procedures which were independently assessed as a summative assessment using the validated competency assessment tool (CAT). Additionally, LAPCO used *global assessment scale (GAS)* forms as a formative tool to assess proficiency-gain and guide when learners are ready for summative assessment. The trainee and trainer could then monitor which areas of the operation or skill they needed to focus on and shorten the learning curve. These assessment tools showed predictive validity. This program is still to be replicated on this scale in other emerging technologies, such as robotic surgery.

Other areas for support to enhance learning include real time feedback and support through telementoring/telestration likened to air traffic controllers in the aviation industry, where a remote surgeon can be supported by a mentor through a procedure.[51,52]

The BAUS curriculum explains that a mentorship program needs to be structured for effective feedback. The mentor must enhance learning through exchange of knowledge, practical learning, and continuous feedback.[25]

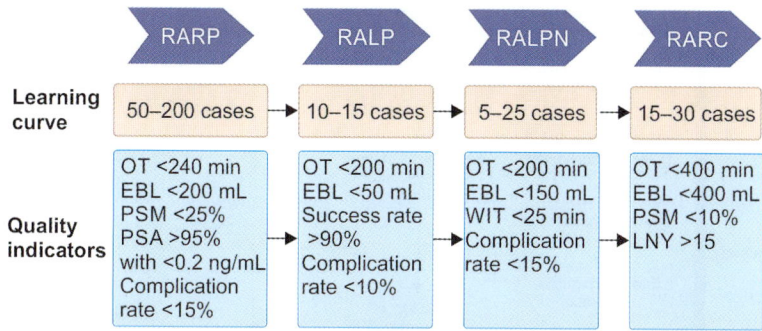

Fig. 2: BAUS "sign-off" recommendations based on current evidence.[25,35] (RARP: robotic-assisted radical prostatectomy; RALP: robot-assisted laparoscopic pyeloplasty; RALPN: robotic-assisted laparoscopic partial nephrectomy; RARC: robotic-assisted radical cystectomy)

This is important to note as effective feedback should be continuous, objective and validated. Currently, most objective tools for robotic surgery skills assessment are summative.

BAUS and NICE note that mentor-/fellowships need to be in high volume centers that are "off" their institutional learning curve.[25] Access to these centers needs to be considered with individual learning curves and standardizing curricula globally, taking into account that there will be geographical variation. **Figure 2** is an example from the BAUS curriculum where there is an opportunity to enhance training through validated formative assessment tools to shorten the learning curve, due to the large volume of caseload considered necessary before sign-off.

Figure 2 shows the expected progression through these procedures, each one from left to right becoming more complex. The lower numbers indicate that once proficient in RARP they would be expected to have a shorter learning curve for the next procedures. Quality indicators seen in **Figure 2** could also have other objective measures related to patient outcome added in formative and summative assessments, including intraoperative error analysis, shown to be directly related to patient outcome in one study looking at rectal cancer surgery.[53]

Global assessment scale forms have been adopted in laparoscopic surgery which could be modified and validated for robotic surgery. Feedback to trainee surgeons could be broken down into a modular pathway **(Fig. 3)** with a CUSUM curve for each part, to highlight which areas of need are greatest, once the proficiency gain curve is at a satisfactory level, already existing summative assessment tools could be used for "sign-off" and accreditation.

Assessment Tools

Assessment is defined as the process of collecting and evaluating information to measure progress. It is established that assessment shapes the experience

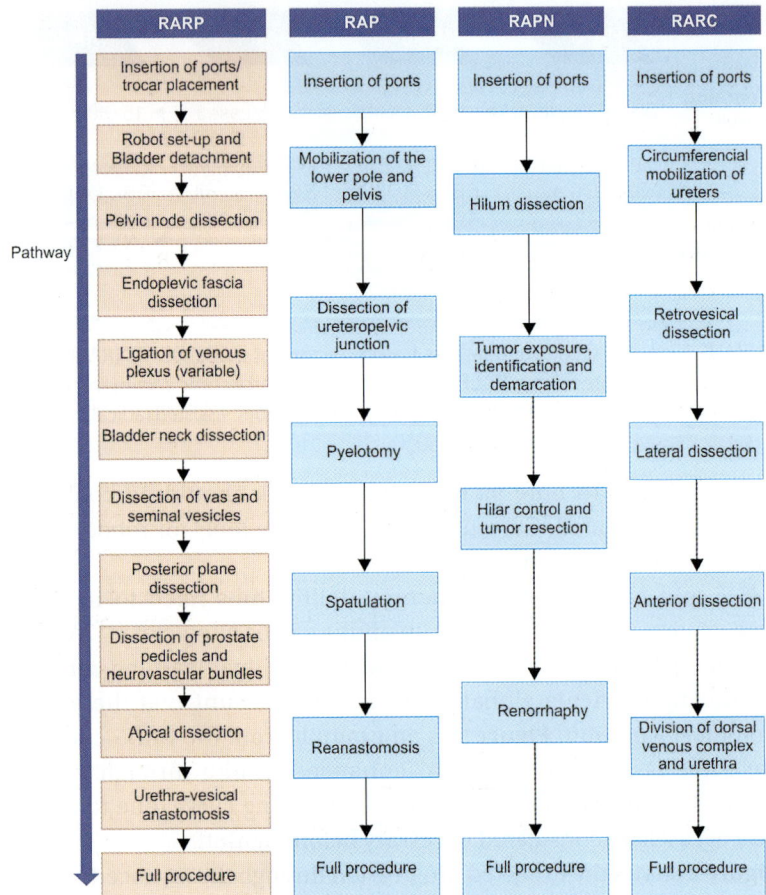

Fig. 3: BAUS modular pathways.[25]

of students and influences their behavior more than any other element of their education.[46] Broad categories of assessment include formative and summative.

Formative Assessment Tools

Formative assessment (FA) is a tool to monitor progress and provide feedback to a student to inform training and education. In other words, it is an assessment for learning. Feedback is shown to raise student achievement; however, quality of feedback is the key.[54] Feedback needs to identify the gap in skills or knowledge, but also advise how to narrow this gap.

To assess and train surgeons to improve; validated, reliable and objective formative assessment tools should be used. Patient outcomes such as morbidity and mortality are often used to assess a surgeon's learning curve. Issues arise here as this does not provide a detailed analysis of operative areas that need improvement,[55] missing a key learning opportunity immediately after the operation.

The UK's LAPCO successfully used and validated GAS forms. These are designed as a type of formative assessment, outlining main operative steps in several procedures. They can be used to see trends and reflect on the degree of independence or competence at each step.[55,56] The main benefits of the form being that it is highly practical and reliable, allowing trainers and trainees to focus on operative steps that need improvement during feedback.

For assessment to be meaningful, therefore, a combination of regular formative assessment with summative assessment at intervals is required.

Global Assessment Scale Tools

In the LAPCO national training program, the GAS forms were found to have construct validity, inter-rater reliability, and internal consistency.[50] They were an integral part of the training pathways, providing a description of individualized proficiency gain curves (CUSUM charts) in terms of the level of support from trainer to trainee required. Using a Juster scale (1-6) at each of the task steps, 5 stating competency, immediate and informative feedback can be given to enhance learning and training, i.e., which area needs the greatest work.

CUSUM charts showed there was a measurable difference between trainees and different steps of the procedure, i.e., the hepatic flexure was the most difficult and theater set up the easiest. The point of upward inflection shows the point at which the trainee scores competency **(Fig. 4)**.

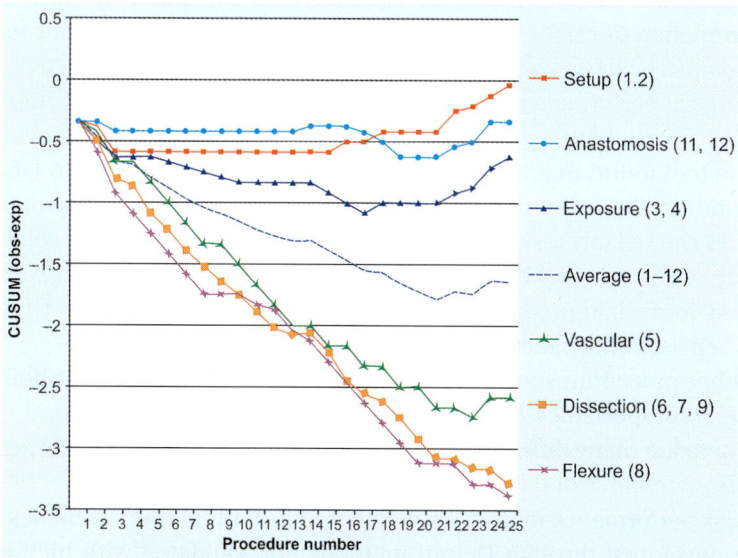

Fig. 4: CUSUM chart for average and specific scores.[55]

Global assessment scale forms are practical, reliable, and valid tools which can be applied to any area of surgery including robotics.

Robotic Summative Assessment Tools

A summative assessment (SA) is an examination or an assessment of learning, i.e., to test a person against a standard or benchmark as to whether they are competent. SA can miss an opportunity to further aid student learning.[44] Types of summative assessment in medical training include multiple choice questions (MCQ), extended matching questions (EMQ) and objective structured clinical examinations (OSCE).

Manual Assessment Tools in Robotic Surgery

A systematic review looked at objective assessment tools of robotic surgery technical skills, all of which are summative assessments, splits in to "manual" and "automatic" assessment. There are several validated, tools have been developed to assess generic skills, including the following:[56]

- *Global Evaluation Assessment of Robotic Skills (GEARS):* Developed from Global Operative Assessment of Laparoscopic Skills (GOALS), it can be used as a formative and summative tool for generic skills.
- *Robotic-Objective Structured Assessment of Technical Skills (R-OSATS):* Developed from OSATS for open and laparoscopic skills.
- *Assessment of Robotic Console Skills (ARCS):* Noted that GEARS did not fully assess independent console skills.

Additionally there are several procedure-specific assessment tools:
- *Observational Clinical Human Reliability Analysis (OCHRA):* It is used for error analysis can be used in conjunction with procedure-specific tools.
- *Competency Assessment Tool (CAT):* It is developed to evaluate technical surgical performance as it has concurrent validity, tested by comparing CAT scores with error analysis using OCHRA. The study developing the tool found that CAT scores were inversely proportional to OCHRA counts,[57] i.e., a better surgical skill score equated to fewer errors. The CAT can reliably assess technical performance in laparoscopic colorectal surgery, which could be adapted by other specialties. In-training GAS and CAT forms had predictive validity in surgical performance after LAPCO when assessing patient outcomes.
- Other procedure-specific tools exist within laparoscopy and robotics in different specialties, e.g., in urology PACE, RACE and CASE.

There are many different tools available and used, however, few actively outside of research and within clinical practice.

Task performance metrics assessment tools for multiple specialties have been developed through Delphi methods and validated with high inter-rater reliability when compared other tools such as GEARS. The conclusion being that they are more objective with binary answers. The tools provide a detailed step-by-step description for the operation, with definitions of errors and critical errors. These tools are promising, however, need to go undergo further evaluation including benchmarking i.e. pass/fail parameters for summative assessment or credentialing of a surgeon as competent.

In an ideal world, an agreed standardized tool would be used for formative and summative assessment, which would be modified for the skill or procedure. Using GEARS as a formative assessment for generic robotic skills and GAS tools for procedure-specific robotic skills are promising.

For summative assessment tools, again GEARS can be used as a generic tool, and CAT could be modified for robotic procedure-specific assessment in conjunction with OCHRA as video error analysis.

Currently, the shortcomings of OCHRAs are—it is manual and incredibly time consuming. The aim would be to create large, video data sets with OCHRA analysis and have machine learning with artificial intelligence to create automatic feedback after an operation to the surgeon.

Automated Assessment Tools in Robotic Surgery

Robotic surgery can provide automatic data for assessment which in the coming years will be developed further, the aim is to have validated and reliable assessment tools which do the same as the manual assessment tools and more, only with instant results. Automated performance metrics (APMs) remove the risk of human bias and are entirely objective theoretically, improving reliability and validity.[56]

Automated performance metrics collected by the da Vinci robot include kinematic instrument tracing, system events such as camera movement, clutch use, third instrument swap and energy, finally surgical video data can be recorded for further analysis. However, they are not used by surgeons routinely or in feedback and training. Intuitive created the dVLogger, which has been likened to a black box recorder within the aviation industry. It allows recording of anonymized video and movement data recording, however, again it is not used routinely for analysis, feedback, and training.

Current APM data collected from robot systems have shown promising ability to distinguish expertise,[58] however, correlation between them and manual assessment has varied among studies.[56] Other disadvantages, currently, include making feedback meaningful from automated data and needing additional devices to record APMs, there are studies underway to analyze their relationship and further develop these tools.[59]

■ ARTIFICIAL INTELLIGENCE

Further evaluation and development are needed within APMs, however, it is an exciting area of robotics particularly with the advent of artificial intelligence in surgery. Deep learning models could drive automation and reinforcement learning of "good" and "not-so-good" outcomes through artificial neural networks.[60] Current research and application within the operative setting is in anatomical and phase recognition, gesture (surgical movement) analysis and application of deep learning to kinematic data which has been able to predict patient outcomes. In order to develop and evaluate deep-learning models further, large annotated datasets need to be made publicly available in open data sets for academic purposes. The goal is to give the surgeon instant, meaningful feedback, e.g., technical performance, visual anatomical queues and possible patient outcomes. This will enhance learning and improve patient care.

■ CONCLUSION

Robotic surgery is widely used across specialties with its use increasing globally, demanding standardization of training, assessment, and the credentialing of safe robotic surgeons.

Currently, assessment tools and curricula are undergoing development and evaluation. Step-by-step training is essential with verified training centers providing validated assessment and credentialing to ensure independent surgical practice is safe with good patient outcomes.

As VR simulation improves so too will access to these platforms and the initial stages of robotic training, as the number of robot-assisted surgical procedures becomes more widespread, so will the need for accredited training centers.

■ REFERENCES

1. Marnoa Private Wealth. Intuitive surgical: A leader in surgical robots. [online] Available from: https://www.fountaingroup.ca/blog/2021/05/10/intuitive-surgical-a-leader-in-surgical-robots?sc_lang=en. [Last Accessed December, 2022].
2. Szold A, Bergamaschi R, Broeders I, Dankelman J, Forgione A, Langø T, et al. European Association of Endoscopic Surgeons (EAES) consensus statement on the use of robotics in general surgery. Surg Endosc. 2015;29(2):253-88.
3. Herron DM, Marohn M. SAGES-MIRA Robotic Surgery Consensus Group. A consensus document on robotic surgery. Surg Endosc. 2008;22(2):313-25; discussion 311-2.
4. Broeders I. Robotics, the next step? Best practice and research. Clin Gastroenterol. 2014;28:225-32.
5. Lee EC, Rafiq A, Merrell R, Ackerman R, Dennerlein JT. Ergonomics and human factors in endoscopic surgery: a comparison of manual vs telerobotic simulation systems," Surg Endosc. 2005;19(8):1064-70.
6. Bagrodia A, Raman JD. Ergonomics considerations of radical prostatectomy: physician perspective of open, laparoscopic, and robot-assisted technique. J Endourol. 2009;23(4):627-33.

7. van der Schatte Olivier RH, Van't Hullenaar CD, Ruurda JP, Broeders IA. Ergonomics, user comfort, and performance in standard and robot-assisted laparoscopic surgery. Surg Endosc. 2009;23(6):1365-71.
8. Byrn JC, Schluender S, Divino CM, Conrad J, Gurland B, Shlasko E, et al. Three-dimensional imaging improves surgical performance for both novice and experienced operators using the da Vinci Robot System. Am J Surg. 2007; 193(4):519-22.
9. Moorthy K, Munz Y, Dosis A, Hernandez J, Martin S, Bello F, et al. Dexterity enhancement with robotic surgery. Surg Endosc. 2004;18(5):790-5.
10. Arezzo A, Vettoretto N, Francis NK, Bonino MA, Curtis NJ, Amparore D, et al. The use of 3D laparoscopic imaging systems in surgery: EAES consensus development conference 2018. Surg Endosc. 2019;33(10):3251-74.
11. Cambridge Dictionary. Dexterity. [online] Available from: https://dictionary.cambridge.org/dictionary/english/dexterity. [Last Accessed December, 2022].
12. Hernandez JD, Bann SD, Munz Y, Moorthy K, Datta V, Martin S, et al. Qualitative and quantitative analysis of the learning curve of a simulated surgical task on the da Vinci system. Surg Endosc. 2004;18(3):372-8.
13. Yohannes P, Rotariu P, Pinto P, Smith AD, Lee BR. Comparison of robotic versus laparoscopic skills: is there a difference in the learning curve? Urology. 2002;60(1):39-45; discussion 45.
14. Brodie A, Vasdev N. The future of robotic surgery. Ann R Coll Surg Engl. 2018; 100(Suppl 7):4-13.
15. Zorn KC, Gautam G, Shalhav AL, Clayman RV, Ahlering TE, Albala DM. Training, credentialing, proctoring and medicolegal risks of robotic urological surgery: recommendations of the society of urologic robotic surgeons. J Urol. 2009; 182:1126-32.
16. Collins JW, Levy J, Stefanidis D, Gallagher A, Coleman M, Cecil T. Utilising the Delphi process to develop a proficiency-based progression train-the-trainer course for robotic surgery training. Eur Urol. 2019;75(5):775-85.
17. Ahmed K, Khan R, Mottrie A, Lovegrove C, Abaza R, Ahlawat R, et al. Development of a standardised training curriculum for robotic surgery: a consensus statement from an international multidisciplinary group of experts. BJU Int. 2015;116(1):93-101.
18. ECRI Institute. (2014). Top 10 Health Technology Hazards for 2015. Health Devices. [online] Available from: https://www.ecri.org/Resources/Whitepapers_and_reports/Top_Ten_Technology_Hazards_2015.pdf. [Last Accessed December, 2022].
19. Collins JW, Wisz P. Training in robotic surgery, replicating the airline industry. How far have we come? World J Urol. 2020;38(7):1645-51.
20. Dixon F, Keeler B. Robotic surgery: training, competence assessment and credentialing. Bull Royal Coll Surg Engl. 2020;102(7):185.
21. Reason J. Human error: models and management. BMJ. 2000;320(7237): 768-70.
22. Fisher RA, Dasgupta P, Mottrie A, Volpe A, Khan MS, Challacombe B, et al. An over-view of robot assisted surgery curricula and the status of their validation. Int J Surg. 2015;13:115-23. [Last Accessed December, 2022].
23. Aggarwal R, Grantcharov TP, Darzi A. Framework for systematic training and assessment of technical skills, J Am Coll Surg. 2007;204(4):697-705.

24. Santok GD, Raheem AA, Kim LH, Chang K, Chung BH, Choi YD, et al. Proctorship and mentoring: its backbone and application in robotic surgery. Investig Clin Urol. 2016;57(Suppl 2):S114-S120.
25. BAUS. Robotic Surgery Curriculum. [online] Available from: https://www.baus.org.uk/professionals/baus_business/publications/83/robotic_surgery_curriculum/. [Last Accessed December, 2022].
26. Veronesi G, Dorn P, Dunning J, Cardillo G, Schmid RA, Collins J, et al. Outcomes from the Delphi process of the Thoracic Robotic Curriculum Development Committee. Eur J Cardiothorac Surg. 2018 1;53(6):1173-9.
27. Ismail A, Wood M, Ind T, Gul N, Moss E. The development of a robotic gynaecological surgery training curriculum and results of a delphi study. BMC Med Educ. 2020;20(1):66.
28. Stolzenburg JU, Qazi HA, Rai BP. The European Association of Urology robotic training curriculum: the journey has only just begun. Eur Urol. 2015;68: 300-1.
29. Andolfi C, Umanskiy K. Mastering robotic surgery: where does the learning curve lead us? J Laparoendosc Adv Surg Tech A. 2017;27:470-4.
30. Tsai A, Osborne A, Welbourn R. Teaching Advanced Laparoscopic Skills in Surgery for Morbid Obesity. In: Training in Minimal Access Surgery. New York: Springer; 2015. pp. 107-27.
31. Francis NK, Fingerhut A, Bergamaschi R, Motson R. Training in Minimal Access Surgery. New York: Springer; 2015.
32. Jiménez-Rodríguez RM, Rubio-Dorado-Manzanares M, Díaz-Pavón JM, Reyes-Díaz ML, Vazquez-Monchul JM, Garcia-Cabrera AM, et al. Learning curve in robotic rectal cancer surgery: current state of affairs. Int J Colorectal Dis. 2016; 31(12):1807-15.
33. Guend H, Widmar M, Patel S, Nash GM, Paty PB, Guillem JG, et al. Developing a robotic colorectal cancer surgery program: understanding institutional and individual learning curves. Surg Endosc. 2017;31(7):2820-8.
34. Sian TS, Tierney GM, Park H, Lund JN, Speake WJ, Hurst NG, et al. Robotic colorectal surgery: previous laparoscopic colorectal experience is not essential. J Robot Surg. 2018;12: 271-7.
35. Abboudi H, Khan MS, Guru KA, Froghi S, de Win G, Van Poppel H, et al. Learning curves for urological procedures: a systematic review. BJU Int. 2014;114(4): 617-29.
36. Sinclair P, Kable A, Levett-Jones T. The effectiveness of internet-based e-learning on clinician behavior and patient outcomes: a systematic review protocol. JBI Database System Rev Implement Rep. 2015;13(1):52-64.
37. Jakimowicz JJ, Buzink S. Training Curriculum in Minimal Access Surgery. In: Training in Minimal Access Surgery. New York: Springer; 2015. pp. 15-34.
38. Abboudi H, Khan MS, Aboumarzouk O, Guru KA, Challacombe B, Dasgupta P, et al. Current status of validation for robotic surgery simulators—a systematic review. BJU Int. 2013;111(2):194-205.
39. Ahmed K, Amer T, Challacombe B, Jaye P, Dasgupta P, Khan MS. How to develop a simulation programme in urology. BJU Int. 2011;108(11):1698-702.
40. Costello DM, Huntington I, Burke G, Farrugia B, O'Connor AJ, Costello AJ, et al. A review of simulation training and new 3D computer-generated synthetic organs for robotic surgery education. J Robot Surg. 2021:1-15.

41. Goh AC, Goldfarb DW, Sander JC, Miles BJ, Dunkin BJ. Global evaluative assessment of robotic skills: validation of a clinical assessment tool to measure robotic surgical skills. J Urol. 2012;187(1):247-52.
42. Schmidt MW, Köppinger KF, Fan C, Kowalewski KF, Schmidt LP, Vey J, et al. Virtual reality simulation in robot-assisted surgery: meta-analysis of skill transfer and predictability of skill. BJS Open. 2021;5(2):zraa066.
43. Seymour NE, Gallagher AG, Roman SA, O'Brien MK, Bansal VK, Andersen DK, et al. Virtual reality training improves operating room performance: results of a randomized, double-blinded study. Ann Surg. 2002;236(4):458-63; discussion 463-4.
44. Issenberg SB, McGaghie WC, Petrusa ER, Lee Gordon D, Scalese RJ. Features and uses of high-fidelity medical simulations that lead to effective learning: a BEME systematic review. Med Teach. 2005;27(1):10-28.
45. Ahmed K, Jawad M, Abboudi M, Gavazzi A, Darzi A, Athanasiou T, et al. Effectiveness of procedural simulation in urology: a systematic review. J Urol. 2011;186(1):26-34.
46. O'Shaughnessy S, Joyce, P. Summative and Formative Assessment in Medicine: the Experience of an Anaesthesia Trainee. Int J High Educ. 2015.
47. Melnyk R, Ezzat B, Belfast E, Saba P, Farooq S, Campbell T, et al. Mechanical and functional validation of a perfused, robot-assisted partial nephrectomy simulation platform using a combination of 3D printing and hydrogel casting. World J Urol. 2020;38(7):1631-41.
48. Ghazi A. A Call for Change. Can 3D Printing Replace Cadavers for Surgical Training? Urol Clin North Am. 2022;49(1):39-56.
49. Kwak JM, Park S. Training for New Techniques and Robotic Surgery in Minimal Access Surgery. In: Training in Minimal Access Surgery. New York: Springer; 2015. pp. 141-50.
50. Hanna GB, Mackenzie H, Miskovic D, Ni M, Wyles S, Aylin P, et al. Lapco program. Laparoscopic Colorectal Surgery Outcomes Improved After National Training Program (LAPCO) for Specialists in England. Ann Surg. 2022;275(6):1149-55.
51. Anvari M, McKinley C, Stein H. Establishment of the world's first telerobotic remote surgical service: for provision of advanced laparoscopic surgery in a rural community," Ann Surg. 2005;241(3):460-4.
52. Sebajang H, Trudeau P, Dougall A, Hegge S, McKinley C, Anvari M. The role of telementoring and telerobotic assistance in the provision of laparoscopic colorectal surgery in rural areas. Surg Endosc. 2006;20(9):1389-93.
53. Curtis NJ, Foster JD, Miskovic D, Brown CSB, Hewett PJ, Abbott S, et al. Association of Surgical Skill Assessment with Clinical Outcomes in Cancer Surgery. JAMA Surg. 2020:e201004.
54. Shepard LA. Commentary: evaluating the validity of formative and interim assessment. Educ Meast Issues Prac. 2009;28(3):32-7.
55. Miskovic D, Wyles SM, Carter F, Coleman MG, Hanna GB. Development, validation and implementation of a monitoring tool for training in laparoscopic colorectal surgery in the English National Training Program. Surg Endosc. 2011;25(4):1136-42.
56. Chen J, Cheng N, Cacciamani G, Oh P, Lin-Brande M, Remulla D, et al. Objective Assessment of Robotic Surgical Technical Skill: A Systematic Review. J Urol. 2019;201(3):461-9.

57. Miskovic D, Ni M, Wyles SM, Kennedy RH, Francis NK, Parvaiz A, et al. National Training Programme in Laparoscopic Colorectal Surgery in England. Is competency assessment at the specialist level achievable? A study for the national training programme in laparoscopic colorectal surgery in England. Ann Surg. 2013;257(3):476-82.
58. Fard MJ, Ameri S, Darin Ellis R, Chinnam RB, Pandya AK, Klein MD. Automated robot-assisted surgical skill evaluation: Predictive analytics approach. Int J Med Robot. 2018;14(1):5.
59. Hung AJ, Chen J, Jarc A, Hatcher D, Djaladat H, Gill IS. Development and Validation of Objective Performance Metrics for Robot-Assisted Radical Prostatectomy: A Pilot Study. J Urol. 2018;199(1):296-304.
60. Bhandari M, Zeffiro T, Reddiboina M. Artificial intelligence and robotic surgery: current perspective and future directions. Curr Opin Urol. 2020;30(1):48-54.

CHAPTER 3

Development of Endoscopic Biliary Surgery Navigated by Artificial Intelligence

Yohei Kono, Masafumi Inomata, Seigo Kitano

■ INTRODUCTION

Artificial intelligence (AI) is a branch of computer science that uses algorithms to approximate human cognitive functions such as problem solving, decision making, object detection, and classification.[1] Deep learning refers to learning using deep neural networks, in which a machine automatically extracts features from data without the need for human intervention, if given a sufficient amount of data. The usefulness of this technology is expected in a variety of medical fields, such as cancer diagnosis in radiological imaging and polyp identification in endoscopy.[2-4] However, the use of real-time surgical navigation is extremely complex, and as it not yet fully understood, deep learning has not yet been demonstrated. Laparoscopic cholecystectomy (LC), which began in the 1980s, is performed in approximately 27,000 cases per year in Japan,[5] and expert surgeons are often required to make difficult intraoperative decisions during the procedure. In fact, the frequency of biliary injury, a serious complication of LC, is 0.6%. In a survey of more than 600 specialists in Asia, including Japan, 72.3% of them reported that they had experienced or almost experienced bile duct injury.[6] Even experienced surgeons are at risk for causing bile duct injury during cholecystectomy, and it has been reported that a common cause of bile duct injury is a simple misconception of the patient's anatomy as perceived by the surgeon.[7-10] In recent years, research and development have been conducted on the use of AI to aid in the safe performance of LC. We have developed an AI system using deep learning to present anatomical landmarks during LC for the purpose of preventing bile duct injury and have conducted validation experiments in a clinical setting. In this report, we review the current status of the application of AI to navigation technology in LC, including the background of our system development.

■ SIGNIFICANCE OF AN ARTIFICIAL INTELLIGENCE NAVIGATION APPLICATION IN LAPAROSCOPIC CHOLECYSTECTOMY

In cholecystectomy, distortion of the anatomical structures due to inflammation or anomaly often results in misconception of the biliary tract, and this misconception must be corrected before the procedure is performed to prevent biliary injury. Surgeons repeatedly use their knowledge and experience to select the optimal procedure according to the transforming conditions of the surgical field during surgery. We believe that "implicit knowledge" is hidden in the surgeon's perceptions, judgments, and actions during surgery, and furthermore, the surgeon's cognition and judgment of the ever-changing situation in the surgical field can prevent misinterpretations of dissection that could lead to bile duct injury. Even among experts, this implicit knowledge varies from person to person, depending on their experience and ability, and thus the risk of medical complications differs. In addition, surgical teams do not always include surgeons with sufficient judgment and extensive experience, and in situations in which surgeons lack the implicit knowledge necessary for successful surgery, the significance of a medical system that compensates for this lack would be high. In our research team, to avoid complications in LC, we extracted teaching data from endoscopic surgeries and trained AI with this implicit knowledge about anatomical landmarks in the important process of "deployment of the Calot's triangle at the neck of the gallbladder." We developed "smart endoscopic surgery," a system through which anatomical landmarks are superimposed on intraoperative endoscopic images by AI. Similar efforts are underway around the world. Madani et al. investigated the use of deep learning in computer vision to identify complex and poorly defined anatomical structures in the surgical field and developed a model. This model performs semantic segmentation functions to identify safe and dangerous zones of dissection and other anatomical structures in LC.[11] Other efforts to assess surgical difficulty include training models to identify inflammation scores defined from gallbladder findings, such as the Parkland scale. This automated assessment may be useful in optimizing workflow in the operating room by predicting surgical progress and providing feedback to the surgeon to promote the mastery of surgical technique.[12,13]

■ ANATOMICAL LANDMARKS TO AVOID BILE DUCT INJURY

In LC, the following anatomic landmarks are emphasized as important to recognize to avoid bile duct injury: (1) the cystic duct, (2) the common bile duct, and (3) the hepatic S4 (left medial segment), which requires safe deployment of the "Calot triangle" composed of these landmarks. In addition, Connor et al. proposed that the surgical field should be safely secured by starting the serosal incision on the gallbladder side at the hypothetical line connecting landmark 4, Rouviere's sulcus, and the inferior margin of the hepatic S4, which is an established technique to be followed, especially in difficult cholecystectomies due to high inflammation.[14] We defined these four structures as anatomical landmarks to avoid bile duct injury and developed a system to intraoperatively display them **(Fig. 1)**. Madani et al. defined the

Development of Endoscopic Biliary Surgery Navigated by Artificial Intelligence

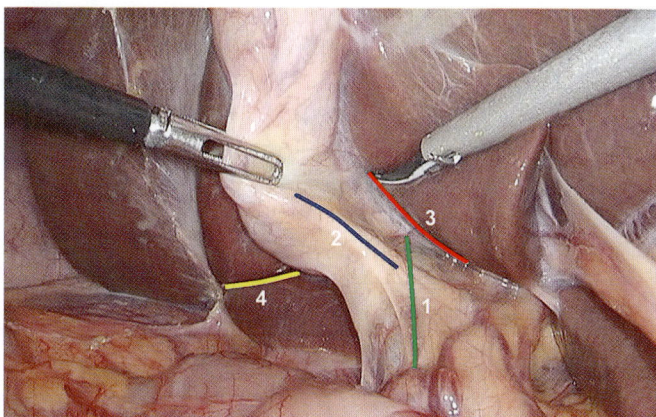

Fig. 1: Anatomical landmarks for laparoscopic cholecystectomy. (1) Common bile duct (2) Cystic duct, (3) Lower edge of hepatic left medial segment (S4), and (4) Rouviere's sulcus.

safe dissection zone (Go zone) as the area within Calot's triangle (near the lower end of the gallbladder) where further dissection is unlikely to cause bile duct injury and is considered safe. The No-Go zone is defined as a deep area within Calot's triangle where further dissection is unnecessary and is considered dangerous due to its high potential to cause bile duct injury. This dangerous zone includes the hepatoduodenal ligament, the hepatic portal region, and all structures below it.[11] Further, Strasberg proposed the concept of the critical view of safety (CVS) to avoid bile duct injury.[15] Mascagni et al.[16] developed a model to evaluate the achievement of the CVS criteria according to Strasberg,[15] which are: (1) two tubular structures connected to the gallbladder should be clearly visible (the two structures criterion), (2) in the deployed Calot's triangle, only the two cystic structures and the cystic plate should be unobstructed (the hepatocystic triangle criterion), and (3) the lower third of the gallbladder is detached from the cystic plate (the cystic plate criterion). They set the CVS criteria as above and showed that it is possible to train the model for the segmentation of these anatomical structures and assessment of the CVS criteria.

■ LANDMARK INDICATION BY ARTIFICIAL INTELLIGENCE

We built an information-rich platform (IRP) development flow for AI landmark indication **(Fig. 2)**. From the videos of LCs performed at our hospital, we excluded videos with noticeable bleeding or videos in which landmarks were not clearly displayed. Then, from the 99 selected videos, we extracted scenes in which Calot's triangle was depicted and created a dataset for deep learning training and for evaluating the estimation accuracy of the training model using an annotation tool that we originally developed. The four landmark-labeled images and the endoscopic image were combined into a dataset. After further rechecking by two other expert endoscopic surgeons,

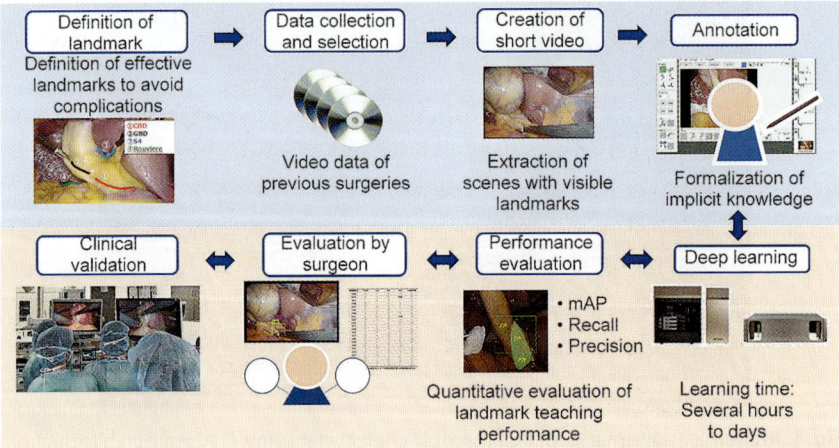

Fig. 2: Information-rich platform (IRP) development.

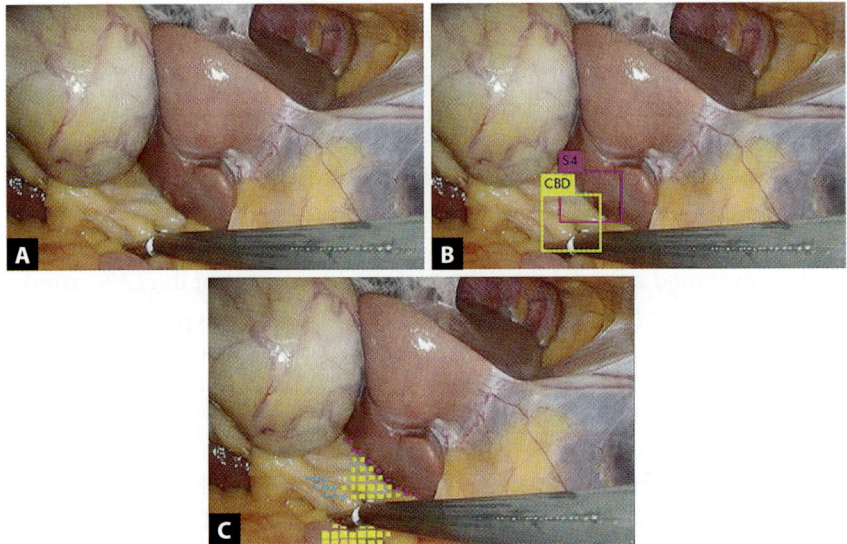

Figs. 3A to C: Landmark indication images. (A) Original image; (B) Rectangle indication image; (C) Tile indication image. (CBD: common bile duct)

we finally labeled the 2,339 images with the segments of 2,119 common bile ducts, 1,895 cholecystic ducts, 2,144 hepatic S4 inferior margins, and 2012 Rouviere's sulci. Of the 99 selected videos, 76 videos were used for deep learning training and 23 for evaluation of estimation accuracy. Because the simultaneous intraoperative display of landmarks requires the landmarks to be displayed without delay, YOLOv3, a fast and accurate detection algorithm, was used to create rectangular or tiled versions of the annotated region display **(Figs. 3A to C)**. Expert endoscopic surgeons evaluated each of the 23 videos for the display of important landmarks in our performance

Development of Endoscopic Biliary Surgery Navigated by Artificial Intelligence

evaluation and found AI landmark indication useful in 95.7% of the cases.[17] Other commonly used indices for performance evaluation include Intersection-Over-Union (IOU) and the Dice/F1 spatial correlation index, which are commonly used in computer vision and measure the overlap between the actual object location area (ground truth) and the predicted area of the object segmented by AI. The ability to correctly or incorrectly classify each pixel in an image relative to a reference (ground truth) is expressed in such normal terms as average accuracy, sensitivity, specificity, negative predictive value, and positive predictive value.[18,19]

■ CLINICAL PERFORMANCE EVALUATION OF A PROTOTYPE

To evaluate the feasibility of an AI surgical support system for LC, a prospective clinical performance study was conducted in 10 LCs performed at our hospital from September 2019 to March 2020. The landmark indicating system was displayed on a separate monitor located in front of the operating table **(Fig. 4)**. The operating surgeon performed the procedure without watching the landmark indicating images, and surgeons who were not participating in the operation evaluated the landmark indicating images as evaluators. The surgical cases included five cases of gallbladder stone disease, four cases of acute cholecystitis, and one case of gallbladder polyp. As a result, the system worked properly, with a time lag of only 0.2 seconds for display of the landmark indicating images, which indicates a display with almost no delay.

Three external evaluators (all board-certified surgeons for endoscopic surgery) were asked to objectively evaluate the landmark indicating system in a clinical performance study, using a 5-point rubric to rate the accuracy of the landmarks indicated by the AI. The results showed that the landmark indicating performance of the AI was satisfactory, with an average of four

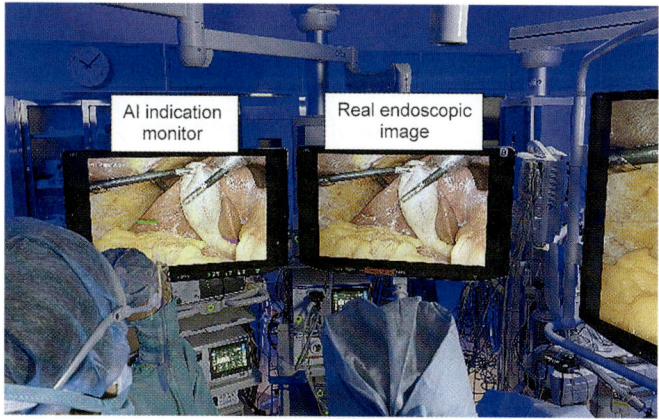

Fig. 4: Clinical validation study of artificial intelligence-navigation laparoscopic cholecystectomy.

or higher, except for the gallbladder duct. In addition, when comparing rectangular and tiled landmarks, tiled landmarks were more easily recognized correctly, which could lead to a reduction in bile duct injury.

CHALLENGES AND IMPROVEMENTS IN THE CLINICAL PERFORMANCE EVALUATION

Although the clinical performance evaluation showed the usefulness of landmark indication, it also revealed several challenges: First, landmarks were misrepresented in surgical phases other than Calot's triangle deployment, which did not require landmark indication. Therefore, we also developed an AI-based surgical phases recognition algorithm to display landmarks only in the appropriate surgical phases. The surgical phases in a standard LC were modified into surgical phases for AI learning that AI can discriminate, and all surgical videos of 115 LC cases performed at our hospital were classified into seven surgical phases (P0-P6) and used for on/off landmark display **(Table 1)**. We created a deep learning model, an image classification algorithm, for 109 cases of teaching data, and evaluated its accuracy using nine untrained cases as test models. The results showed a high average accuracy of 97%.[20] This automatic surgical phase recognition has been reported in several surgical video analysis studies in which AI has been applied and has achieved high accuracy in various fields such as gynecological surgery, colectomy, and sleeve gastrectomy, as well as LC,

TABLE 1: Definition of the surgical phases from Phase 0 to Phase 6.

Phase	Task	Start–end point	Landmark identification
Phase 0	Other	Extracorporeal procedure	Off
Phase 1	Preparation	Lifting the GB—completing clearance around the GB	On
Phase 2	Calot's triangle dissection	Incision of the GB neck—achievement of CVS	On
Phase 3	Clipping and cutting	Insertion of a clipping device—completion of cutting of the cystic duct and artery	Off
Phase 4	Gallbladder (GB) dissection	Dissection of the GB from the liver bed—release of the GB from the liver bed	Off
Phase 5	GB retrieval	Insertion of a retrieval bag—removal of the bag	Off
Phase 6	Cleaning and coagulation	Insertion of a suction device—removal of the device	Off

(CVS: critical view of safety)

in which the difficulty of the surgery varies depending on the degree of inflammation and the time required for each phase is likely to change.[21-25]

The second challenge was that the detection rate of landmarks decreased in cases in which high inflammation or excessive fat was identified. The reason for the lower detection rate was the lack of training data for such cases. However, in cases with high inflammation, even skilled physicians may have difficulty recognizing landmarks as implicit knowledge. Therefore, we are using data expansion techniques to reproduce the inflammatory findings of the gallbladder in noninflammatory cases. By creating pseudo-generated images with abnormal findings of acute cholecystitis and improving the deep learning model to include the pseudo-generated teaching data, we expect that correct landmarks will be indicated even for acute cholecystitis.

■ CONCLUSION

Artificial intelligence development in LC is progressing by repeatedly creating an experimental model, identifying issues through clinical performance evaluations, and overcoming challenges. In addition to landmark indication, we would like to further improve the accuracy of the AI surgical support system that visualizes implicit knowledge by incorporating the newly developed recognition of the surgical phases and response to highly difficult cases into the experimental model. By improving the surgeon's recognition of landmarks, we hope to create a system that will contribute to reducing bile duct injuries in LC.

■ REFERENCES

1. Yu KH, Beam AL, Kohane IS. Artificial intelligence in healthcare. Nat Biomed Eng. 2018;2(10):719-31.
2. McKinney SM, Sieniek M, Godbole V, Godwin J, Antropova N, Ashrafian H, et al. International evaluation of an AI system for breast cancer screening. Nature. 2020;577(7788):89-94.
3. Esteva A, Kuprel B, Novoa RA, Ko J, Swetter SM, Blau HM, et al. Dermatologist-level classification of skin cancer with deep neural networks. Nature. 2017;542(7639):115-8.
4. Berzin TM, Topol EJ. Adding artificial intelligence to gastrointestinal endoscopy. Lancet. 2020;395(10223):485.
5. Inomata M, Shiroshita H, Uchida H, Bandoh T, Akira S, Yamaguchi S, et al. Current status of endoscopic surgery in Japan: The 14th National Survey of Endoscopic Surgery by the Japan Society for Endoscopic Surgry. Asian J Endosc Surg. 2020;13(1):7-18.
6. Iwashita Y, Hibi T, Ohyama T, Umezawa A, Takada T, Strasberg SM, et al. Delphi consensus on bile duct injuries during laparoscopic cholecystectomy: an evolutionary cul-de-sac or the birth pangs of a new technical framework? J Hepatobiliary Pancreat Sci. 2017;24(11):591-602.
7. Giger UF, Michel JM, Opitz I, Th Inderbitzin D, Kocher T, Krähenbühl L, et al. Risk factors for perioperative complications in patients undergoing

laparoscopic cholecystectomy: analysis of 22,953 consecutive cases from the Swiss Association of Laparoscopic and Thoracoscopic Surgery database. J Am Coll Surg. 2006;203(5):723-8.
8. Harboe KM, Bardram L. The quality of cholecystectomy in Denmark: outcome and risk factors for 20,307 patients from the national database. Surg Endosc. 2011;25(5):1630-41.
9. Navez B, Ungureanu F, Michiels M, Claeys D, Muysoms F, Hubert C, et al. Surgical management of acute cholecystitis: results of a 2-year prospective multicenter survey in Belgium. Surg Endosc. 2012;26(9):2436-45.
10. Davidoff AM, Pappas TN, Murray EA, Hilleren DJ, Johnson RD, Baker ME, et al. Mechanisms of major biliary injury during laparoscopic cholecystectomy. Ann Surg. 1992;215:196-202.
11. Madani A, Namazi B, Altieri MS, Hashimoto DA, Rivera AM, Pucher PH, et al. Artificial intelligence for intraoperative guidance: Using semantic segmentation to identify surgical anatomy during laparoscopic cholecystectomy. Ann Surg. 2020;276(2):363-369.
12. Ward TM, Hashimoto DA, Ban Y, Rosman G, Meireles OR. Artificial intelligence prediction of cholecystectomy operative course from automated identification of gallbladder inflammation. Surg Endosc. 2022;36(9):6832-40.
13. Korndorffer JR Jr, Hawn MT, Spain DA, Knowlton LM, Azagury DE, Nassar AK, et al. Situating artificial intelligence in surgery: a focus on disease severity. Ann Surg. 2020;272(3):523-8.
14. Connor SJ, Perry W, Nathanson L, Hugh TB, Hugh TJ. Using a standardized method for laparoscopic cholecystectomy to create a concept operation-specific checklist. HPB (Oxford). 2014;16(5):422-9.
15. Strasberg S. Avoidance of biliary injury during laparoscopic cholecystectomy. J Hepatobiliary Pancreat Surg. 2002;9:543-7.
16. Mascagni P, Vardazaryan A, Alapatt D, Urade T, Emre T, Fiorillo C, et al. Artificial intelligence for surgical safety: Automatic assessment of the critical view of safety in laparoscopic cholecystectomy using deep learning. Ann Surg. 2022;275(5):955-61.
17. Tokuyasu T, Iwashita Y, Matsunobu Y, Kamiyama T, Ishikake M, Sakaguchi S, et al. Development of an artificial intelligence system using deep learning to indicate anatomical landmarks during laparoscopic cholecystectomy. Surg Endosc. 2021;35(4):1651-8.
18. Rezatofighi, Tsoi N, Gwak JY, Sadeghian A, Reid I, Savarese S. Generalized intersection over union: a metric and a loss for bounding box regression. In Proceedings of the IEEE/CVF Conference on Computer Vision and Pattern Recognition. 2019.
19. Sudre CH, Li W, Vercauteren T, Ourselin S, Jorge Cardoso M. Generalised dice overlap as a deep learning loss function for highly unbalanced segmentations. Deep Learn Med Image Anal Multimodal Learn Clin Decis Support (2017). 2017;2017:240-8.
20. Shinozuka K, Turuda S, Fujinaga A, Nakanuma H, Kawamura M, Matsunobu Y, et al. Artificial intelligence software available for medical devices: Surgical phase recognition in laparoscopic cholecystectomy. Surg Endosc. 2022;36(10):7444-52.
21. Hashimoto DA, Rosman G, Witkowski ER, Stafford C, Navarette-Welton AJ, Rattner DW, et al. Computer vision analysis of intraoperative video: Automated

recognition of operative steps in laparoscopic sleeve gastrectomy. Ann Surg. 2019;270(3):414-21.
22. Meeuwsen FC, van Luyn F, Blikkendaal MD, Jansen FW, van den Dobbelsteen JJ. Surgical phase modelling in minimal invasive surgery. Surg Endosc. 2019;33(5):1426-32.
23. Kitaguchi D, Takeshita N, Matsuzaki H, Takano H, Owada Y, Enomoto T, et al. Real-time automatic surgical phase recognition in laparoscopic sigmoidectomy using the convolutional neural network-based deep learning approach. Surg Endosc. 2020;34(11):4924-31.
24. Cheng K, You J, Wu S, Chen Z, Zhou Z, Guan J, et al. Artificial intelligence-based automated laparoscopic cholecystectomy surgical phase recognition and analysis. Surg Endosc. 2022;36(5):3160-8.
25. Bar O, Neimark D, Zohar M, Hager GD, Girshick R, Fried GM, et al. Impact of data on generalization of AI for surgical intelligence applications. Sci Rep. 2020;10(1):22208.

CHAPTER 4

Machine Learning: Does it Prognosticate Colorectal Anastomotic Outcome?

Raj Nagarkar, Yasam Venkata Ramesh

Abstract

Artificial intelligence (AI) research has contributed substantially to the resolution of a variety of healthcare problems, with potential applications in both basic and clinical cancer research. In AI, machine learning (ML) has garnered increasing attention over time in assessing both preoperative and postoperative complications, especially in colorectal cancer (CRC) patients, where ML predictive models have helped clinicians to make effective and accurate decisions by predicting the most common postoperative complications such as colorectal anastomotic leaks (AL) and its related morbidity and mortality based on the patient's history. ML also helps in predicting clinically relevant outcomes such as prognosis, survival, disease-free survival, response to therapy, and relapse. In this chapter, we discuss the potential use of ML algorithm in the preoperative assessment of patients and their prognosis in CRC surgery, the current issues, and limitations.

Keywords: Machine learning, prediction, surgical outcomes, colorectal cancer, anastomotic leakage, clinical prognosis, complications.

■ INTRODUCTION

In the last two decades, cancer research has evolved at an exponential rate with the advent of modern technology. A huge data was being available at the fingertips without processing and giving no conclusion to the medical research community. Such huge data can be a boon in developing sophisticated disease-predicting tools using artificial intelligence (AI), where the data can be analyzed and predicted to derive the outcome of the patients by identifying the similar patterns that happened earlier. Accuracy and disease diagnosis are one of the most challenging and interesting tasks for physicians, where AI can be a helping hand by simulating human intelligence.

These AI systems have three major qualities: adaptability, intelligence, and intentionality. AI systems often incorporate: AI, machine learning (ML), and deep learning (DL) to create a sophisticated intelligence machine that will perform given human functions well **(Fig. 1)**.[1]

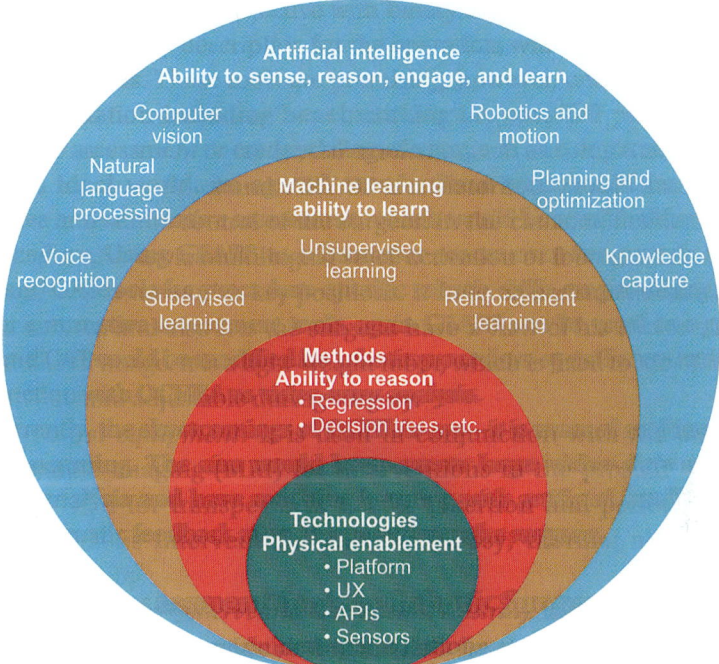

Fig. 1: A visual classification and explanation of AI, ML, and DL. (AI: artificial intelligence; APIs: application programming interfaces; DL: deep learning; ML: machine learning; UX: user experience)
Source: Adapted from Bohnhoff T. (2019).[1]

■ ARTIFICIAL INTELLIGENCE

Artificial intelligence is a field of research in which computers are applied to accomplish tasks by mimicking human intelligence as shown in **Figure 2**.[2-5] AI is broadly classified into three types: artificial super intelligence, artificial general intelligence (AGI, strong AI), and artificial narrow intelligence (ANI, weak or narrow AI). AI-powered medical technologies have been met with enthusiasm because of their 4P model of medicine (Participatory, Personalized, Preventive, and Predictive). AI is being used in health care in various areas such as electronic health records, operation notes, clinical data, genetic diagnosis, electrodiagnosis, laboratory data, diagnostic imaging, mass screening, and records from wearable devices.[2-4,6-13] Food and Drug Administration (FDA) approved several AI-based algorithms and digital tools, such as pain management and psychiatric disorders, virtuality–reality continuum tools for surgery, and surgical navigation systems for computer-assisted surgery, are already available and serving in the market.[9,14-17]

The problems that are best suited for AI technology to solve are:
- *Repetitive tasks:* Manual tasks that follow logical steps to lead to a conclusion

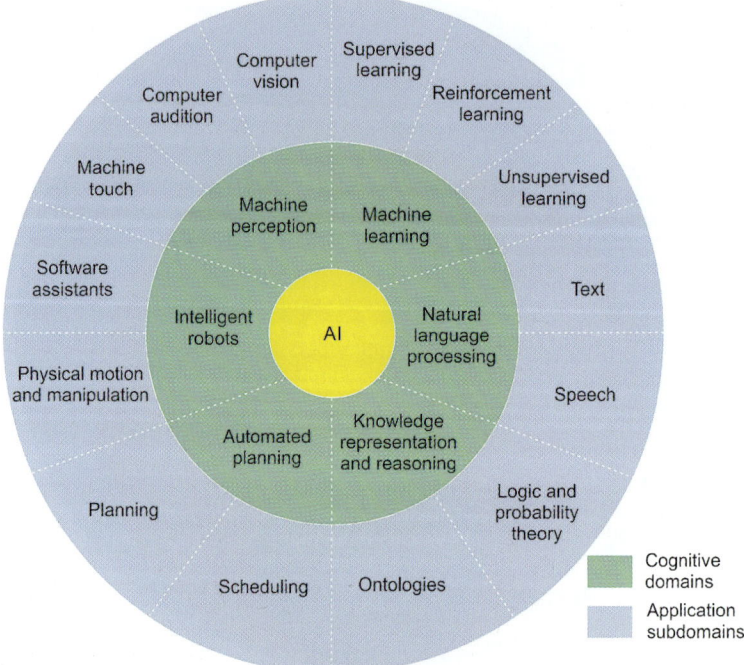

Fig. 2: Artificial intelligence (AI) and its application in various domains.
Source: Adapted from Pathania S. (2019).[5]

- *Data intensive tasks:* Tasks involving analyzing large amounts of data looking for patterns and anomalies
- *Super human tasks:* Tasks that require superhuman capabilities and speak to the limitations of human sensory skills and fine motor skills. (For example: Robotic surgeons can use the most precise movements to perform noninvasive surgeries, and finely tuned computer vision can spot tumors on a magnetic resonance imaging (MRI) when human eyes cannot see it).

■ MACHINE LEARNING

Machine learning is a subfield of AI in which statistical and mathematical approaches are applied to improve the performance of computers. ML helps in predicting the future or classifying the information to help people in making necessary decisions. ML algorithms are trained over instances or examples through which they learn from past experiences and also analyze the historical data. Therefore, as it trains over the examples, again and again, it is able to identify patterns in order to make predictions about the future **(Fig. 3)**.

For nearly 20 years, ML is used in cancer detection and research in the form of decision trees (DTs) and artificial neural networks (ANNs).[18,19] ML has made great advances in the healthcare, biotech, and pharmaceutical

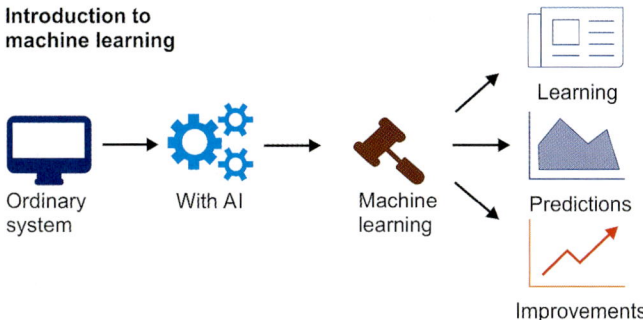

Fig. 3: Schema of machine learning. (AI: artificial intelligence)

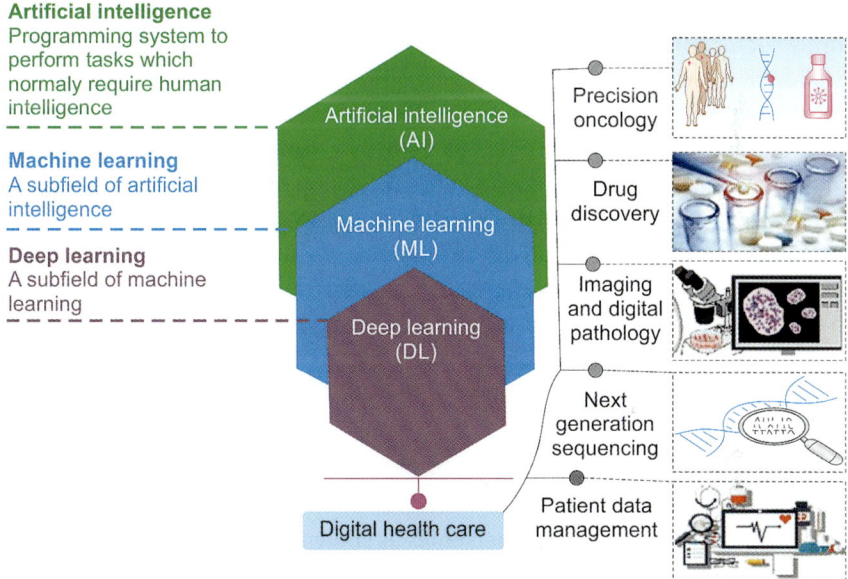

Fig. 4: Applications of AI, ML, and DL in digital health care and oncology to solve healthcare issues and predict optimal treatment outcome.
Source: Adapted from Iqbal MJ et al. (2021).[20]

industries in terms of diagnosing diseases, drug development, individualized precision medicine, and improvement in gene editing **(Fig. 4)**.[20]

Here we discuss it in terms of healthcare and medical field applications, where ML is helping in multiple ways in terms of AI-assisted image analysis for radiology [computed tomography (CT) scans, MRI, ultrasounds, positron emission tomography (PET) scans, and mammography—to identify multiple ailments], MRI-guided biopsies, machine vision for diagnosis and surgery, a war against antibacterial super-resistance, building intelligence into medical devices, clinical workflow optimization, intelligent personal health records, AI-enabled clinical decision support (CDS) systems, guiding population-level disease prevention, improving pathologists' ability to diagnose tissue samples, predictive analytics for hospital resource optimization, cardiac MRI images, and electrocardiograms (to identify and assess the risk of heart-related diseases), skin images (to classify skin lesions), and eye images (to detect diabetic retinopathy and other eye-related ailments), etc.[11,12]

Machine learning is proven to be highly efficient in high-resolution CT (HRCT) and CT machines to diagnose, classify, detect, or distinguish tumors and other malignancies.[21-24] In recent times, researchers have started using ML toward cancer prediction, prognosis, and as an aid in clinical decision-making prior to surgeries for better outcomes,[7,25] where ML first helps in classifying cancer patients into high- or low-risk groups and provides information about its possible progression and subsequent clinical management. A variety of ML tools and techniques are applied to draw such conclusions in cancer research. Such tools include DTs, support vector machines, Bayesian networks, and ANNs for the development of predictive models **(Box 1)**. Overall, all these tools help results in effective and accurate decision-making. In a study conducted by Kourou et al., various ML techniques employed in the modeling of cancer progression and prognosis were reviewed, where such techniques were identified to be highly promising for inference in the cancer domain.[25] In another study by Gonçalves et al., postoperative complications were predicted in cancer patients.[26]

In general, all these AI systems require continuous training data procured from clinical studies.

Such data employed can broadly be classified into two types: training data and test data.[13,14]

Types of Machine Learning

Further, ML is classified into three types as shown in **Figure 5**:[10,27-29]

- *Supervised learning*: Learns by using labeled data, e.g., risk evaluation, forecast sales

BOX 1: Overview of artificial intelligence in healthcare and challenges in obtaining and using data.

Sources of data:	*Types of data employed:*	*Common tools employed:*
• Electronic health records	• Test data	• Hidden Markov model
• Operation notes	• Training data	• Neural network
• Clinical data	*Fields in which used successfully:*	• Support vector machine
• Genetic diagnosis	• Neurology	• Discriminant analysis
• Electrodiagnosis	• Internal medicine	• Random forest decision trees
• Laboratory data	• Clinical pharmacology	• Nearest neighbor analysis
• Diagnostic imaging	• Ophthalmology	• Decision tree analysis
• Mass screening	• Cardiology	• Naïve Bayes
• Records from wearable devices	• Oncology	• Logistic regression
	• Radiology	• Linear regression

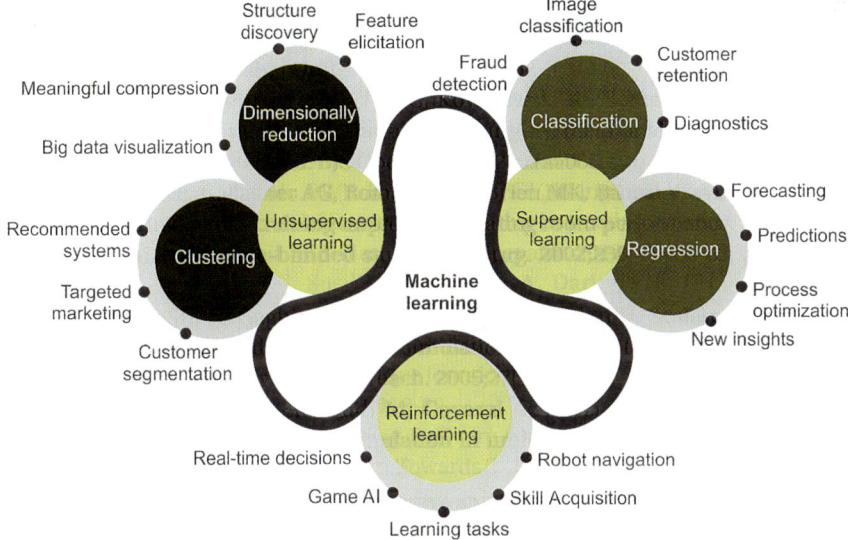

Fig. 5: Different machine learning types and their application. (AI: artificial intelligence)
Source: Adapted from Krzyk K. (2018).[29]

- *Classification:* Where output variable is a category, e.g., "disease"/"no disease"
    - Naïve Bayes classifier
    - Support vector machines
    - Logistic regression
- *Regression:* Where output variable is a real continuous value, e.g., stock price prediction
    - Linear regression
    - Nonlinear regression
    - Bayesian linear regression
- *Unsupervised learning:* Trained using unlabeled data without any guidance, e.g., recommendation system and anomaly detection
    - *Clustering:* Unveiling the inherent groupings in the data, such as grouping animals based on some characteristics/features, e.g., the number of legs
    - *Association:* Discovering association rules such as people that buy X also tend to buy Y.
    Some examples of models that belong to this family are the following:
        - K—means clustering
        - Neural networks
        - Principal component analysis
- *Reinforcement learning*: Works on predefined data interacting with the environment, e.g., self-driving cars, gaming, and healthcare
    - Exploitation or exploration

ARTIFICIAL INTELLIGENCE AND COLORECTAL CANCER

Over 10 million cancer deaths were reported in 2020 alone.[30] The most common cancers in terms of causing death were reported to be lung (1.80 million deaths), colon and rectum (935,000 deaths), and liver (830,000 deaths). The most top three common cancers in terms of new cases of cancer were identified to be breast (2.26 million cases), lung (2.21 million cases), and colorectal (1.93 million cases).[31]

Further, we discuss only colorectal cancer (CRC), the third most commonly occurring cancer in men and the second most commonly occurring cancer in women.[30,32,33] Overall, CRC ranks third in terms of incidence, but second in terms of mortality.[33]

After CRC surgery, the risk of developing procedure-specific complications such as anastomotic leak (AL) was reported to be common. To overcome such complications, ML-based algorithms were used preoperatively to estimate and predict the risk of developing anastomotic insufficiency after colon and colorectal surgery with high accuracy.

Despite a plethora of published data, accurate personalized prediction of AL remains notoriously difficult.[34] Currently, AL risk assessment is done altogether based on the risk factors, experience, and published data. However, such assessments were proven to be highly inaccurate and inadequate.

Partly in response to this, AI and its subset ML have gained momentum to develop risk prediction algorithms and innovative tools to quantify the risk of AL in individual patients. ML was also reported to be helpful in developing precision medicine and the best treatment strategy for different individual patients. Therefore, the application of ML algorithms without depending on the independent risk factors can be much helpful in developing a predictive model for individual decision making.[35] Modern ML techniques have also proven themselves by improving and proving their prognosis accuracy by 15–20%.[25,36]

Compared to classic prognostication systems, ML approaches are "highly beneficial when the target predictive task is fundamentally nonlinear, being able to learn models from multicolinear variables with complex interdependencies."[26] The number of studies/papers related to this matter was also reported to be steadily increased over the years, as shown in **Figure 6**.[26]

Surgical procedures involved in these complicated CRCs are majorly classified into four types:[37]
- Resection and anastomosis
- Resection and stoma
- Diverting loop colostomy without resection
- Sole biopsy.

Colorectal surgeries form a significant core of general surgery, in both elective and emergency settings. Despite improved surgical techniques and perioperative management, postoperative complications such as (AL, 5–15%

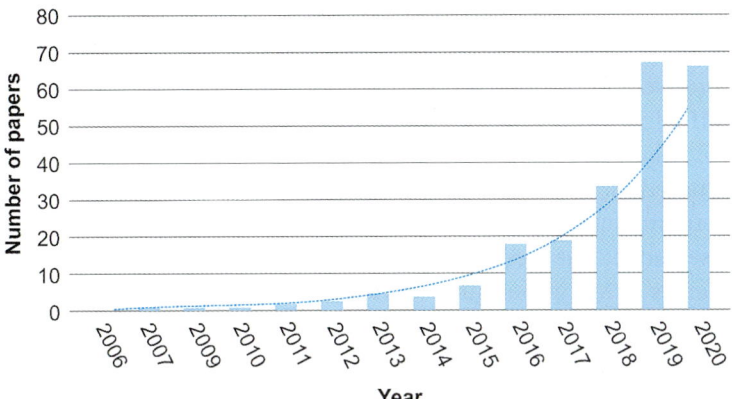

Fig. 6: Number of papers published per year: keyword search "machine learning" and "cancer surgical risk" on PubMed.
Source: Adapted from Gonçalves DM et al. (2021).[26]

of all treated patients) are still high resulting in prolonged hospitalization (≥12 days), readmissions, unplanned return to operation theater, unplanned critical care need, delaying postoperative therapy among those with cancer, increased medical costs/mental trauma, morbidity, and mortality.[34,35,38-41]

Although the rigorous anastomotic operation is an essential measure to prevent AL, its occurrence is still highly unpredictable and largely varies due to the heterogeneity of individual patients.[35] Possible risk factors to look out for in patients are smoking, obesity, cardiovascular disease, prognostic nutritional index, and anemia. Still as of date, accurate risk calculation of AL for individual patients has proven to be a great challenge for both clinicians and surgeons, respectively.[35,42,43]

Many studies have practically proven the negative effect of these risk factors on a patient's overall prognosis. For example, Silber et al.[44] demonstrated the major change in patients' prognosis after the first postoperative complication, even seemingly mild ones. Dorcaratto et al. have studied and concluded the negative effect of the postoperative complications on disease-free survival, overall survival, and recurrence after surgical resection.[45] Merath et al. also confirmed the interaction of complications in a synergistic manner developing into more than one complication, increasing the risk of death exponentially, rather than in an additive way.[41]

To stratify the patient's risk of postoperative morbidity and mortality, multiple risk stratification and predictive tools/models have been proposed such as Physiologic and Operative Severity Score for the Enumeration of Mortality and Morbidity (POSSUM), American Society of Anesthesiologists (ASA) score, and the American College of Surgeons Surgical Risk Calculator (ACS-SRC).[46-48] However, reports from these predictive tools were proven to be moderately predictive with limited clinical applicability.[49-51]

To overcome their limitations, AI and ML tools have become largely famous because of their accuracy in predicting the risk and assessing the preoperative and postoperative clinical outcomes.[26,36,41,52,53] Nartowt et al. used ML algorithms and identified an effective mass screening method for CRC risk in large populations using only personal health data.[53] Julian et al. studied the clinical outcomes of CRC using ML, where the outcomes that were predicted with the highest accuracies were radio chemotherapy response and relapse (yes/no), as well as disease-free survival and survival.[36]

In terms of ML in postsurgical risk analysis, Gonçalves et al. reported it as an area still in its infancy and its success is highly dependent on the multidisciplinary collaborations between data scientists and health professionals.[26] In another study by Merath et al., the ML algorithm was found to have a good predictive ability in identifying the occurrence of any postoperative specific complications with a C-statistic of 0.74, outperforming the ACS-SRC (C-statistic 0.71) and ASA (C-statistic 0.58).[41] Cristina et al. also predicted postoperative complications using ML statistical models—kernel methods and heterogeneous clinical data to make a framework for preoperative clinical decision support. Findings from their study have suggested that blood tests and vital signs data can give an early warning to improve the AL diagnosis, hence providing the basis for alerting clinicians about patients at risk for complications, so that appropriate actions can be taken.[54] In another study by Wen et al., ML-based random forest algorithm was used in AL prediction, where they concluded that their prediction model is more accurate and has been demonstrated to have better performance in the prediction of AL after anterior resection for rectal cancer.[55] Sammour et al. also studied the use of AI analytics to predict the AL after colon cancer surgery using the Binational Colorectal Cancer Audit registry and retrospective data of 9 years. Results from their study are in favor of using an AL risk calculator prior to surgery to predict AL.[34] A large observational clinical trial [prediction of anastomotic insufficiency risk after colorectal surgery – (PANIC)] is being conducted by Anas Taha et al., where ML-based application is used to accurately predict the patients at risk for AL.[38] Reports from this large clinical data of estimated 11,000 participants with a follow-up of 5 years were expected to be completed by 2022.

LIMITATIONS AND POTENTIAL ISSUES WITH ARTIFICIAL INTELLIGENCE

- Current supervised learning through the input of data should be replaced with unsupervised learning.
- Most of the data procured is from single-center retrospective studies, with possible selection bias.
- Lack of external validation on center, type of data, and their method of collection

- Data variability due to voluntary contribution and data privacy legislation of different states/countries
- Prospective data from multiple centers that share the universal language should be used to improve data specificity, sensitivity, overfitting, spectrum bias, and real-time decision-making.
- Uniform universal protocols, outcome reporting tools, and universally linked servers should be developed to avoid substandard data with no important outcomes.
- Tackling the black box problem

CONCLUSION

The current development of ML-based high-performance models based on clinical preoperative and intraoperative variables can be highly beneficial. They can help in predicting and identifying the high-risk AL patients with high accuracy in prior, which in turn will help and improve the clinician's/surgeon's decision-making throughout the process (preoperative and perioperative). However, large multicenter prospective studies are warranted for high specificity and sensitivity to predict the risk of AL in patients. Given how rapidly the field of AI and its evolvement in cancer science, agreeing upon uniform regulatory frameworks of outcome reporting with basic quality standards can revolutionize AI in oncology in the coming decade.

REFERENCES

1. Bohnhoff T. (2019). A Five-Minute Guide to Artificial Intelligence. [online] Available from: https://medium.com/appanion/a-five-minute-guide-to-artificial-intelligence-c4262be85fd3 [Last accessed December, 2022].
2. Bali J, Bali O. Artificial intelligence applications in medicine: a rapid overview of current paradigms. EMJ Innov. 2020;4(1):73-81.
3. Rajkomar A, Dean J, Kohane I. Machine learning in medicine. N Engl J Med. 2019;380(14):1347-58.
4. Shimizu H, Nakayama KI. Artificial intelligence in oncology. Cancer Sci. 2020;111(5):1452-60.
5. Pathania S. (2019). An Introduction to the World of AI. [online]. Available from: https://sumeetpathania2003.medium.com/introduction-to-the-world-of-ai-b07c4c2d3307 [Last accessed December, 2022].
6. Ahmad Z, Rahim S, Zubair M, Abdul-Ghafar J. Artificial intelligence (AI) in medicine, current applications and future role with special emphasis on its potential and promise in pathology: present and future impact, obstacles including costs and acceptance among pathologists, practical and philosophical considerations. A comprehensive review. Diagn Pathol. 2021;16(1):24.
7. National Cancer Institute. (2020). Artificial Intelligence—Opportunities in Cancer Research. [online]. Available from: https://www.cancer.gov/research/areas/diagnosis/artificial-intelligence [Last accessed December, 2022].
8. Hamamoto R, Suvarna K, Yamada M, Kobayashi K, Shinkai N, Miyake M, et al. Application of artificial intelligence technology in oncology: towards the establishment of precision medicine. Cancers. 2020;12(12):3532.

9. Briganti G, Le Moine O. Artificial Intelligence in Medicine: Today and Tomorrow. Front Med (Lausanne). 2020;7:27.
10. Wu J. (2021). AI, Machine Learning, Deep Learning Explained Simply. Towards Data Science. [online] Available from: https://towardsdatascience.com/.
11. Top 10 AI Applications in Healthcare & the Medical Field - dynam. AI [online] Available from: https://www.dynam.ai/
12. Schmitt M. (2021). Artificial Intelligence in Medicine. [online]. Available from: https://www.datarevenue.com/en-blog/artificial-intelligence-in-medicine [Last accessed December, 2022].
13. Cirillo D, Núñez-Carpintero I, Valencia A. Artificial intelligence in cancer research: learning at different levels of data granularity. Mol Oncol. 2021;15(4):817-29.
14. Malloy KM, Milling LS. The effectiveness of virtual reality distraction for pain reduction: a systematic review. Clin Psychol Rev. 2010;30(8):1011-8.
15. Mishkind MC, Norr AM, Katz AC, Reger GM. review of virtual reality treatment in psychiatry: evidence versus current diffusion and use. Curr Psychiatry Rep. 2017;19(11):80.
16. Tepper OM, Rudy HL, Lefkowitz A, Weimer KA, Marks SM, Stern CS, et al. Mixed reality with hololens: where virtual reality meets augmented reality in the operating room. Plast Reconstr Surg. 2017;140(5):1066-70.
17. Overley SC, Cho SK, Mehta AI, Arnold PM. Navigation and robotics in spinal surgery: where are we now? Neurosurg. 2017;80(3S):S86-99.
18. Maclin PS, Dempsey J, Brooks J, Rand J. Using neural networks to diagnose cancer. J Med Syst. 1991;15(1):11-9.
19. Simes RJ. Treatment selection for cancer patients: application of statistical decision theory to the treatment of advanced ovarian cancer. J Chronic Dis. 1985;38(2):171-86.
20. Iqbal MJ, Javed Z, Sadia H, Qureshi IA, Irshad A, Ahmed R, et al. Clinical applications of artificial intelligence and machine learning in cancer diagnosis: looking into the future. Cancer Cell Int. 2021;21(1):270.
21. Dettling M. BagBoosting for tumor classification with gene expression data. Bioinformatics. 2004;20(18):3583-93.
22. Zhou X, Liu KY, Wong ST. Cancer classification and prediction using logistic regression with Bayesian gene selection. J Biomed Inform. 2004;37(4):249-59.
23. Bocchi L, Coppini G, Nori J, Valli G. Detection of single and clustered microcalcifications in mammograms using fractals models and neural networks. Med Eng Phys. 2004;26(4):303-12.
24. Petricoin EF, Liotta LA. SELDI-TOF-based serum proteomic pattern diagnostics for early detection of cancer. Curr Opin Biotechnol. 2004;15(1):24-30.
25. Kourou K, Exarchos TP, Exarchos KP, Karamouzis MV, Fotiadis DI. Machine learning applications in cancer prognosis and prediction. Comput Struct Biotechnol J. 2015;13:8-17.
26. Gonçalves DM, Henriques R, Costa RS. Predicting postoperative complications in cancer patients: a survey bridging classical and machine learning contributions to postsurgical risk analysis. Cancers (Basel). 2021;13(13):3217.
27. Data Flair. (2021). Machine Learning Tutorial – All the Essential Concepts in Single Tutorial. [online] Available from: https://data-flair.training/blogs/machine-learning-tutorial/ [Last accessed December, 2022].

28. Patel A. (2018). Machine Learning Algorithm Overview. [online]. Available from: https://medium.com/ml-research-lab/machine-learning-algorithm-overview-5816a2e6303 [Last accessed December, 2022].
29. Krzyk K. (2018). Coding Deep Learning For Beginners. [online] Available from: https://towardsdatascience.com/coding-deep-learning-for-beginners-types-of-machine-learning-b9e651e1ed9d [Last accessed December, 2022].
30. World Health Organization. Cancer Today. Volume 418, Cancer Today. 1984. [online] Available from: https://gco.iarc.fr/today/home [Last accessed December, 2022].
31. World Health Organization. (2022). Cancer. [online] Available from: https://www.who.int/news-room/fact-sheets/detail/cancer [Last accessed December, 2022].
32. Ferlay J, Soerjomataram I, Dikshit R, Eser S, Mathers C, Rebelo M, et al. Cancer incidence and mortality worldwide: sources, methods and major patterns in GLOBOCAN 2012. Int J Cancer. 2015;136(5):E359-86.
33. Sung H, Ferlay J, Siegel RL, Laversanne M, Soerjomataram I, Jemal A, et al. Global cancer statistics 2020: GLOBOCAN estimates of incidence and mortality worldwide for 36 cancers in 185 countries. CA Cancer J Clin. 2021;71(3):209-49.
34. Sammour T, Cohen L, Karunatillake AI, Lewis M, Lawrence MJ, Hunter A, et al. Validation of an online risk calculator for the prediction of anastomotic leak after colon cancer surgery and preliminary exploration of artificial intelligence-based analytics. Tech Coloproctol. 2017;21(11):869-77.
35. Shao S, Liu L, Zhao Y, Mu L, Lu Q, Qin J. Application of machine learning for predicting anastomotic leakage in patients with gastric adenocarcinoma who received total or proximal gastrectomy. J Pers Med. 2021;11(8):748.
36. Gründner J, Prokosch HU, Stürzl M, Croner R, Christoph J, Toddenroth D. Predicting clinical outcomes in colorectal cancer using machine learning. Stud Health Technol Inform. 2018;247:101-5.
37. Menegozzo CAM, Teixeira-Júnior F, Couto-Netto SDD, Martins-Júnior O, Bernini CO, Utiyama EM. Outcomes of elderly patients undergoing emergency surgery for complicated colorectal cancer: a retrospective cohort study. Clinics (Sao Paulo). 2019;74:e1074.
38. Anas Taha, Stephanie TM, Ahmad H, Tobias S, Michel A. The Prediction of Anastomotic Insufficiency Risk After Colorectal Surgery (PANIC) Study: Development and External Validation of an International, Multicenter Machine Learning Algorithm for Prediction of Anastomotic Insufficiency After Colonic or Colorectal Anastomosis. [online] Available from: https://clinicaltrials.gov/ProvidedDocs/81/NCT04985981/Prot_001.pdf [Last accessed December, 2022].
39. Hosaka H, Takeuchi M, Imoto T, Yagishita H, Yu A, Maeda Y, et al. Machine learning-based model for predicting postoperative complications among patients with colonic perforation: a retrospective study. J Anus Rectum Colon. 2021;5(3):274-80.
40. Elfanagely O, Toyoda Y, Othman S, Mellia JA, Basta M, Liu T, et al. Machine learning and surgical outcomes prediction: a systematic review. J Surg Res. 2021;264:346-61.
41. Merath K, Hyer JM, Mehta R, Farooq A, Bagante F, Sahara K, et al. Use of machine learning for prediction of patient risk of postoperative complications after liver, pancreatic, and colorectal surgery. J Gastrointest Surg. 2019;24(8):1843-51.2

42. Oshi M, Kunisaki C, Miyamoto H, Kosaka T, Akiyama H, Endo I. Risk factors for anastomotic leakage of esophagojejunostomy after laparoscopy-assisted total gastrectomy for gastric cancer. Dig Surg. 2018;35(1):28-34.
43. Gong W, Li J. Combat with esophagojejunal anastomotic leakage after total gastrectomy for gastric cancer: A critical review of the literature. Int J Surg. 2017;47:18-24.
44. Silber JH, Rosenbaum PR, Trudeau ME, Chen W, Zhang X, Kelz RR, et al. Changes in prognosis after the first postoperative complication. Med Care. 2005;43(2):122-31.
45. Dorcaratto D, Mazzinari G, Fernandez M, Muñoz E, Garcés-Albir M, Ortega J, et al. Impact of postoperative complications on survival and recurrence after resection of colorectal liver metastases: systematic review and meta-analysis. Ann Surg. 2019;270(6):1018-27.
46. Copeland GP, Jones D, Walters M. POSSUM: a scoring system for surgical audit. Br J Surg. 1991;78(3):355-60.
47. Gawande AA, Kwaan MR, Regenbogen SE, Lipsitz SA, Zinner MJ. An Apgar score for surgery. J Am Coll Surg. 2007;204(2):201-8.
48. Bilimoria KY, Liu Y, Paruch JL, Zhou L, Kmiecik TE, Ko CY, et al. Development and evaluation of the universal ACS NSQIP surgical risk calculator: a decision aid and informed consent tool for patients and surgeons. J Am Coll Surg. 2013;217(5):833-42.e1-3.
49. Sahara K, Paredes AZ, Merath K, Tsilimigras DI, Bagante F, Ratti F, et al. Evaluation of the ACS NSQIP surgical risk calculator in elderly patients undergoing hepatectomy for hepatocellular carcinoma. J Gastrointest Surg. 2019;24(3):551-9.
50. Gleeson EM, Shaikh MF, Shewokis PA, Clarke JR, Meyers WC, Pitt HA, et al. WHipple-ABACUS, a simple, validated risk score for 30-day mortality after pancreaticoduodenectomy developed using the ACS-NSQIP database. Surg. 2016;160(5):1279-87.
51. Beal EW, Saunders ND, Kearney JF, Lyon E, Wei L, Squires MH, et al. Accuracy of the ACS NSQIP online risk calculator depends on how you look at it: results from the united states gastric cancer collaborative. Am Surg. 2018;84(3):358-64.
52. Ng ZQ, Jung JK, Theophilus M. Artificial intelligence in pre-operative assessment of patients in colorectal surgery. Turk J Color Dis. 2021;32:99-104.
53. Nartowt BJ, Hart GR, Muhammad W, Liang Y, Stark GF, Deng J., et al. Robust Machine learning for colorectal cancer risk prediction and stratification. Front Big Data. 2020;3:6.
54. Soguero-Ruiz C, Hindberg K, Mora-Jiménez I, Rojo-Álvarez JL, Skrøvseth SO, Godtliebsen F, et al. Predicting colorectal surgical complications using heterogeneous clinical data and kernel methods. J Biomed Inform. 2016;61:87-96.
55. Wen R, Zheng K, Zhang Q, Zhou L, Liu Q, Yu G, et al. Machine learning-based random forest predicts anastomotic leakage after anterior resection for rectal cancer. J Gastrointest Oncol. 2021;12(3):921-32.

CHAPTER 5

Precision Surgery in Rectal Resection Using Hyperspectral Imaging and Fluorescence Angiography

Jignesh Gandhi, Amay Banker

■ INTRODUCTION

Colorectal cancer is the third most common cancer worldwide.[1] Surgery remains the cornerstone of treatment in these patients. Technological advancements in and refinement of diagnostic procedures, minimal access surgery and perioperative chemotherapy have gradually improved long-term outcomes in rectal cancer over the past two decades.

We have also seen repeated validation of minimal access surgery with multiple randomized trials demonstrated similar oncological outcomes in patients with colon cancer after laparoscopic surgery when compared with traditional open procedures.[2-4] Laparoscopic colorectal surgery is associated with lesser postoperative pain, an early return of gut function and a shorter hospital stay when compared with open surgery and is now considered the standard of care by many.[2-5]

One of the main drawbacks of the laparoscopic approach is the absence of tactile feedback during surgery.[6] This makes tissue recognition difficult, especially when performing a total mesorectal excision in a deep and narrow pelvis in patients with rectal cancer. Ultimately, this increases the technical complexity of the procedure and therefore the risk of compromising the oncological resection. So, technological advances which would help the surgeon delineate the tumor from surrounding normal tissue would greatly safeguard radical resection margins.

Erguner et al. suggested that totally laparoscopic surgery avoids ischemia-reperfusion of the colon during extracorporeal anastomosis. Safe specimen extraction site such as the Pfannenstiel incision would lead to fewer adhesions, and better cosmesis.[7] However, an increased reliance on energy devices for bowel division, lack of tactile feedback, and interposition of a vision system between the surgeon and the tissues impair the judgement of the surgeon while evaluating the bowel edge perfusion during intracorporeal suturing of the colon.[8] More sophisticated technologies like Doppler ultrasound, and oxygen spectroscopy are thought to be reliable methods to evaluate organ perfusion. However, a lack of reproducibility, the high costs, and the need for technical expertise restricts the use of these newer technologies.[9]

Fluorescence imaging using indocyanine green (ICG) dye has been used earlier to visualize the perfusion of tissues in open surgery. The same technology has been adapted for use in laparoscopy, allowing real-time assessment of organ perfusion based on the detection of fluorescence emitted by ICG when these perfused tissues are exposed to near-infrared (NIR) light.

In this chapter, we will discuss two technological advances which help overcome some limitations of the laparoscopic approach for colorectal malignancy—(1) Use of ICG fluorescence angiography (FA) to evaluate bowel perfusion and (2) Hyperspectral imaging (HSI) as a tool to distinguish tumor from healthy colorectal tissue ensuring radical margins.

■ INDOCYANINE GREEN FLUORESCENCE ANGIOGRAPHY

In the 1970s ophthalmologists first used ICG to visualize choroidal circulation.[10] Plastic and reconstructive surgeons later demonstrated that areas of inadequate tissue perfusion and potential tissue breakdown could be identified via perfusion mapping by ICG-FA.[11,12] Kudszus et al. pioneered the use of ICG to evaluate intestinal perfusion at the time of colorectal resections.[13] Subsequent researchers demonstrated a 12% reduction in the rates of anastomotic leaks when ICG was used intraoperatively to assess perfusion of the resected margins.[14] So, fluorescence imaging has emerged as an aid to decide the extent of resections in colorectal malignancies.

Properties of Indocyanine Green

Indocyanine green is a tricarbocyanine dye, which is stable at room temperature and is soluble in water.[15] While in the plasma, ICG binds strongly to plasma proteins and remains exclusively within the intravascular compartment. With its short half-life of 3–5 minutes, ICG also allows for repeated evaluations during the same surgical procedure, which is not possible with other dyes such as fluorescein. ICG does not have any known metabolites, and it is rapidly excreted by the liver into bile. It has a safe pharmacological profile with very low adverse reaction rates: 0.05% risk of severe reactions.[16] ICG absorbs light in the NIR spectrum with the maximum absorption at 805 nm. The use of this excitation light induces fluorescence from the ICG, which is maximum at 835 nm **(Fig. 1)**. This fluorescence of ICG operates in the so-called "*tissue optical window*," that is, the NIR light used for excitation of ICG, and its fluorescence penetrates the tissue up to a depth of 5 mm, which allows us to observe the deeper vascular structures accurately.[17-20]

Available Systems for Indocyanine Green Fluorescence Angiography

Several fluorescent angiography systems are available for laparoscopic as well as open surgery, including the Stryker 1588 AIM Platform (Portage,

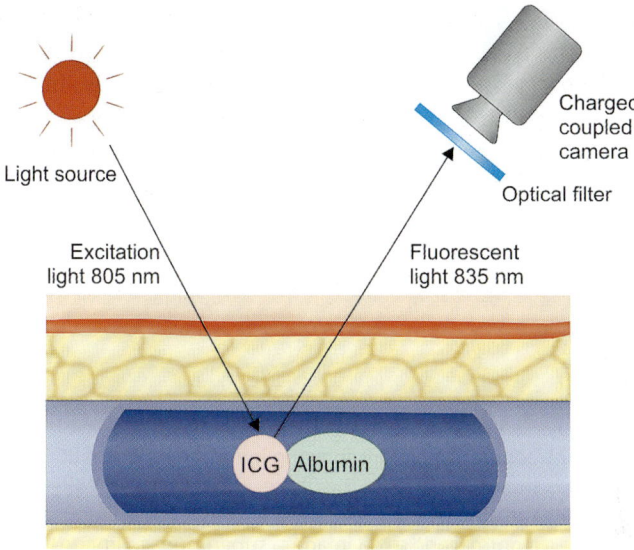

Fig. 1: A schematic diagram showing the working of an indocyanine green (ICG) fluorescent system. The ICG molecule bound to albumin remains in the intravascular compartment. When excited by an "excitation light" it fluoresces at a maximum of 835 nm which can be captured by a camera system.

MI, USA), PINPOINT (Novadaq, Mississauga, ON, Canada), D-Light NIR/ICG (Karl Storz, Tuttlingen, Germany), IC-View (Pulsion Medical Systems, Munich, Germany), PDE-neo System (Hamamatsu Photonics, Hamamatsu, Japan), the SPY Elite Kit (LifeCell Corporation, Bridgewater, NJ, USA), and the da Vinci Firefly robotic surgical system (Intuitive Surgical, Sunnyvale, CA, USA). These systems function as a conventional laparoscope in white light mode but can be used for ICG-FA by activating the NIR imaging mode, in which ICG is visualized as white fluorescence on a black background.[21] Some systems have a mechanism where the illumination is rapidly alternated between white light and NIR light with the two images rapidly processed and superimposed. The result is a laparoscopic image under regular illumination with an overlay of color-graded fluorescence. This composite image provides greater information than either white light or fluorescence imaging alone and does not require the surgeon to keep switching between modes during the operation **(Figs. 2A to D)**.

Fluorescence Angiography to Assess Anastomoses Perfusion

Anastomotic leaks remain the most dreaded complication after colorectal surgery. Despite improvements in understanding of bowel physiology, better surgical energy devices, and advancements in laparoscopic equipment, the rates of anastomotic leaks have remained fairly consistent, occurring in 3–20% of the patients undergoing colorectal resections.[22] Inadequate blood

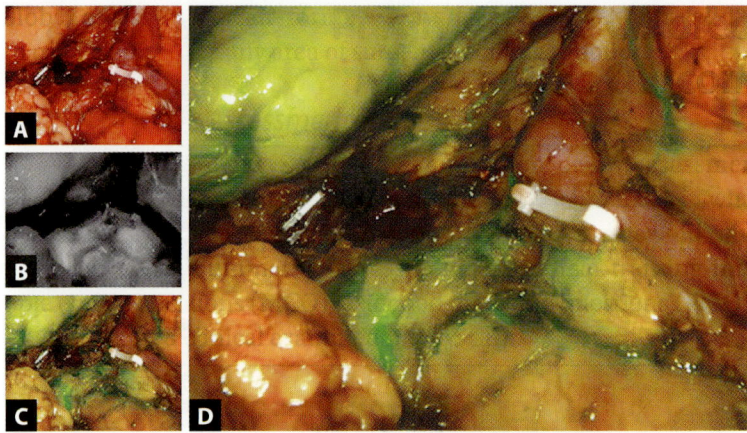

Figs. 2A to D: An intraoperative picture showing indocyanine green (ICG) fluorescence. The normal image is shown as part A of the figure. A near-infrared (NIR) image is shown in part B where only the area where there is ICG fluorescence is illuminated. By rapidly alternating between a normal and a NIR image, a superimposed image is created which is shown as part C and part D.

flow at resection margins has been touted as one of the main reasons for anastomotic leaks. At present, the adequacy of perfusion at resection margins is confirmed by palpable pulses, lack of bowel discoloration, and pulsatile bleeding at cut ends of the anastomoses. The high leak rates suggest that this clinical assessment alone is not reliable, even in open surgery. The inability to assess some of these factors in laparoscopic surgery further limits the surgeon. ICG-FA can aid intraoperative decision making by visualizing bowel perfusion in real time. For detection of bowel vascularity, 5 mg ICG diluted in normal saline is injected intravenously followed by a 10-cc saline flush. After intravenous injection, the ICG which finds its way into tissues is excited by using an NIR light source. The induced fluorescence from the ICG is captured by the NIR camera. This enables the surgeon to assess the vascularity of the cut bowel edges in real time.

There is growing body of evidence, which suggests intraoperative assessment of perfusion affects patient outcomes, including the incidence of anastomotic leaks in colorectal surgery.[13,14,17,21,23-29] Boni et al. reported the results of 107 laparoscopic colorectal resections in which fluorescence showed an insufficiently perfused bowel margin in 4 of 107 patients. These were subsequently revised prior to anastomosis, and no patient suffered an anastomotic leak.[17] In 2016, Degett et al. performed a systematic review of 10 cohort studies including 916 patients and reported that intraoperative fluorescent angiography was associated with a reduced risk of anastomotic leaks {3 of 693 patients; 3.3% [95% confidence interval (CI) 1.97–4.63]} when compared with routine assessment without fluorescent angiography [19 of 223 patients; 8.5% (4.8–12.2)].[30]

The PILLAR-II (Perfusion Assessment in Laparoscopic Left-sided/Anterior Resection) trial was a prospective, multicenter, clinical trial performed at 11 centers across the USA, done to assess the role of perfusion assessment via fluorescence imaging. 139 patients who underwent a left hemicolectomy and/or an anterior resection had perfusion assessments done in this trial. The use of FA influenced a change in the operative plan in 11 (8%) of the 139 patients. The overall incidence of anastomotic leakage was 1.4%. Notably, none of the patients where the resection margins were altered based on FA suffered a leak.[31] Although the existing body of literature is promising, we await data from the ongoing PILLAR-III trial which is a multicentric, randomized controlled trial to define the role of FA in routine clinical practice.

Ureter Visualization using Indocyanine Green Fluorescence Angiography

Iatrogenic ureteric injury is relatively uncommon after colorectal surgery. However, a higher incidence is reported with laparoscopic colorectal surgery, especially in low anterior resections.[32] Preoperative ureteric stenting for intraoperative identification comes with an additional cystoscopic procedure and its associated costs, which increases operative times and possibly, the length of hospital stay.[33] ICG fluorescence of the ureters has value for facilitating their identification, especially in minimally invasive colorectal surgery. ICG reversibly binds to the urothelial lining of the ureters enabling visualization of the ureter by a NIR camera. Since ICG operates within the optical tissue window, it can be used to track the entire course of the ureters, even when obscured by fibrotic tissue. Full-thickness ureteric injuries can be easily identified by observing the leak of ICG into the surgical field.

Endoscopic Tattooing of Colorectal Lesions

Precise localization of colorectal lesions can directly affect recurrence and survival. India ink is the standard marking dye used for endoscopic tattooing, but complications such as perforation, peritonitis, abscesses, and adhesion-associated ileus limit its use.[34] ICG has been recently used by many researchers to guide colorectal resections.[35-38] In these reports, peritumoral injection of ICG to identify the lesion was found to be safe, feasible, and effective. Nagata et al. performed a comparative study between India Ink and ICG for tattooing early colorectal lesions. They endoscopically injected 24 patients with both ICG and India ink at separate sites 4 days before laparoscopic colorectal surgery. The authors found that the NIR fluorescence showed tumor location clearly and accurately in 100% of patients, whereas 10 of 24 patients had negative staining of India ink. The site of ICG injection did not show signs of inflammation, fibrosis, or necrosis, whereas the India ink injection sites had edema, vasculitis, necrosis, and microabscess formation within the resected bowel wall.[39]

Sentinel Lymph Node Mapping

In oncological resections, sentinel lymph node mapping allows targeted identification and harvesting of potentially metastatic lymph nodes, which has the potential to change the operative course and recommendations for adjuvant therapy postoperatively. ICG is emerging as a powerful tool for lymphatic mapping, and identification of the sentinel node in colorectal cancer. NIR fluorescence mapping of the pelvic sidewall in low rectal cancer can guide the need for extended lymphadenectomy in appropriate patients, and spare tumor negative sentinel node patients from the morbidity of a lateral pelvic sidewall nodal dissection.[40,41] Cahill and colleagues used ICG fluorescence for real-time identification of lymphatic drainage and sentinel mesocolic lymph nodes in 18 patients who underwent laparoscopic colorectal surgery. The authors found that the fluorescence helped to identify the sentinel nodes within the specimen or outside the standard resection field prior to formal dissection, and was able to guide their management. In this series, mesocolic sentinel lymph nodes were identified outside the traditional resection field in four of 18 patients using ICG fluorescence.[38]

■ HYPERSPECTRAL IMAGING IN COLORECTAL CANCER

The lack of tactile feedback during laparoscopic surgery makes the tumor recognition difficult. This can be a contributor to R1 resections, particularly for the distal margins in rectal cancer. Hence, alternative techniques that enable the surgeon to distinguish tumor from normal tissue during minimally invasive surgery would be of great benefit to ensure adequate resection. HSI is emerging as a tool to ensure negative margins in these circumstances, distinguishing tumor from healthy colorectal tissue.

Hyperspectral Imaging

In HSI, a broadband light source is used to illuminate an object. The light interacts with the tissue undergoing reflection, scattering, and absorption of its photons. This interaction is dependent on tissue characteristics. After several interactions within the tissue, part of the light is reflected back onto the surface of the tissue which is detected by the hyperspectral camera. In the resulting hyperspectral image, the tissue specific spectral changes of the light can be analyzed. By combining two-dimensional spatial data with a third spectral dimension, the system generates a three-dimensional data cube called a "hypercube".[42] The spatial information of HSI images shows the size and shape of target tissue, while the spectral information reveals composition-specific information. At the margins of a tumor, the spectral properties of tissues change and can be appreciated using a hyperspectral camera. Although the resolution and spectral properties of HSI are outstanding, the Achilles heel of this technology is the imaging depth. Light entering tissues is scattered, reflected, and absorbed; therefore, it has a limit of optical penetration.[43-45] The optical penetration depth varies with tissue composition and wavelength and only reaches millimeter level depths in tissues. Currently in vivo tumor detection by HSI is mainly focused on exterior organs, or organs that can be reached via endoscopy, or laparoscopy. HSI has been mainly applied in two areas: (1) Tissue differentiation (2) Perfusion assessment.

Tissue Recognition using Hyperspectral Imaging

Hyperspectral imaging has the potential to differentiate accurately between tissue types in a contrast-free and noninvasive manner. Theoretically, it is an ideal intraoperative tool which should help identify pathological tissues or essential anatomical structures in the surgical field. As mentioned previously, HSI captures information in the form a data "hypercube" the details of which are beyond the scope of this chapter. Once this information is captured, various machine learning algorithms have been devised that can promptly differentiate between different tissues, based on their spectral characteristics. Jansen-Winkeln et al. were able to discriminate colorectal cancer from healthy tissue with a good degree of precision (sensitivity 86%, specificity 95%) using HSI combined with artificial neural networks. Additionally, other spectral differences, reflecting variations in concentrations of oxygenated hemoglobin or water content, were detected. Interestingly, these variations were related to important oncologic characteristics, such as local tumor extension or previous neoadjuvant chemotherapy.[46]

The oncologic procedures are increasingly performed using minimally invasive platforms in colorectal cancers. Currently, no reliable HSI system suitable for minimally invasive surgery is available because of the steep increase in costs to miniaturize the HSI unit. Further research at this frontier of surgery may potentially lead to the use of HSI to assess tumor behavior, and the efficacy of a neoadjuvant treatment. This would open new therapeutic strategies, possibly involving individualized treatment strategies.

Perfusion Assessment

Along with ICG-FA, HSI imaging represents another objective method of assessing bowel perfusion in real time with the potential to reduce the incidence of postoperative leaks. In a pioneer study, Akbari et al. created a small bowel ischemia model in a pig and by using a custom-made HSI system were able to detect bowel ischemia.[47] Inspired by this study, Kulcke researched application of HSI for perfusion mapping using a compact spatial scanner HSI camera. This camera had a short acquisition time (<10 s) and provided a quantitative heatmap of several physiological parameters, such as tissue oxygen saturation (StO_2), near-infrared perfusion index (NIR PI), and tissue water index (TWI), thanks to their proprietary algorithms.[48] Using these indices they were able to measure the relative oxygen level of the blood and the distribution of water and hemoglobin content in the recorded area. However, their solution was cumbersome and was difficult to use in routine surgical practice. In 2019, advances in HSI technology made hyperspectral cameras suitable for clinical use, and studies emerged which demonstrated that determination of the resection margin by HSI was possible and it provided the surgeon with an objective aid for assessment of the bowel perfusion and ideal anastomotic area in colorectal surgery.[49] Jansen-Winkeln and associates compared the use of ICG-FA and HSI in a nonrandomized, prospective study in 32 consecutives cases of colorectal surgery. They found that the resection line had to be converted to a better perfused area in 33% of the cases. The authors mentioned that ICG-FA had a faster image acquisition time for the first image, but the surgeon had to wait for 5 minutes or more for repeated images. HSI could be performed repeatedly since there were no image artifacts from a previously injected dye. Ultimately, they reported that both methods provided similar results in determining the perfusion border.[50]

Literature suggests HSI could successfully identify ischemic bowel segments and quantify bowel perfusion. While ICG fluorescence has found a foothold in open and laparoscopic colorectal surgery, the exact role of HSI is yet to be determined. While several experimental forays into these technologies have been referenced above, their low sample sizes indicate that these are niche, early endeavors. Larger randomized trials are required to understand the clinical value of HSI-based systems for intraoperative assessment of bowel perfusion and its impact on outcomes after colorectal resections.

■ CONCLUSION

Indocyanine green fluorescence and HSI are promising tools that can help decide the extent of resections colorectal surgery with the aim to reduce postoperative leaks and ensure adequacy of oncologic resection. Although FA was initially introduced as a tool to assess anastomotic perfusion, its applications continue to evolve. Our literature review shows that these are safe, feasible, and fairly reliable techniques with minimal adverse effects and can be used in a broad array of colorectal procedures. While we await randomized controlled trials to define the standards and protocols for use, FA continues to have a considerable clinical benefit in minimally invasive colorectal surgery.

Hyperspectral imaging allows for analysis of the tissue chemical composition at a molecular level and virtually in real time. Early applications of the technology have shown great promise and HSI-based tissue recognition systems continue to evolve. Current research is aimed to produce HSI systems capable of quantifying perfusion in tissues and tissue recognition algorithms, which will be integrated as a part of the precision surgery operating room.

■ REFERENCES

1. Ferlay J, Soerjomataram I, Dikshit R, Eser S, Mathers C, Rebelo M, et al. Cancer incidence and mortality worldwide: sources, methods and major patterns in GLOBOCAN 2012. Int J Cancer. 2015;136(5):E359-86.
2. Bonjer HJ, Hop WCJ, Nelson H, Sargent DJ, Lacy AM, Castells A, et al. Laparoscopically assisted vs open colectomy for colon cancer: a meta-analysis. Arch Surg. 2007;142(3):298-303.
3. Keller DS, Jenkins CN. Safety with Innovation in Colon and Rectal Robotic Surgery. Clinics in colon and rectal surgery. 2021;34(5):273-9.
4. Liang Y, Li G, Chen P, Yu J. Laparoscopic versus open colorectal resection for cancer: A meta-analysis of results of randomized controlled trials on recurrence. European J Surg Oncol. 2008;34(11):1217-24.
5. Pascual M, Salvans S, Pera M. Laparoscopic colorectal surgery: Current status and implementation of the latest technological innovations. World J Gastroenterol. 2016;22(2):704.
6. Ottermo MV, Øvstedal M, Langø T, Stavdahl Ø, Yavuz Y, Johansen TA, et al. The role of tactile feedback in laparoscopic surgery. Surgical laparoscopy, endoscopy & percutaneous techniques. 2006;16(6):390-400.
7. Erguner I, Aytac E, Baca B, Hamzaoglu I, Karahasanoglu T. Total laparoscopic approach for the treatment of right colon cancer: a technical critique. Asian J Surg. 2013;36(2):58-63.
8. Su H, Wu H, Bao M, Luo S, Wang X, Zhao C, et al. Indocyanine green fluorescence imaging to assess bowel perfusion during totally laparoscopic surgery for colon cancer. BMC Surg. 2020;20(1):1-7.
9. Klein KU, Stadie A, Fukui K, Schramm P, Werner C, Oertel J, et al. Measurement of cortical microcirculation during intracranial aneurysm surgery by combined laser-Doppler flowmetry and photospectrometry. Neurosurgery. 2011;69(2):391-8.
10. Flower RW, Hochheimer BF. Clinical infrared absorption angiography of the choroid. Am J Ophthalmol. 1972;73(3):458-9.
11. Holm C, Tegeler J, Mayr M, Becker A, Pfeiffer UJ, Mühlbauer W. Monitoring free flaps using laser-induced fluorescence of indocyanine green: A preliminary experience. Microsurgery. 2002;22(7):278-87.
12. Still J, Law E, Dawson J, Bracci S, Island T, Holtz J. Evaluation of the circulation of reconstructive flaps using laser induced fluorescence of indocyanine green. Ann Plast Surg. 1999;42(3):266-74.
13. Kudszus S, Roesel C, Schachtrupp A, Höer JJ. Intraoperative laser fluorescence angiography in colorectal surgery: a noninvasive analysis to reduce the rate of anastomotic leakage. Langenbecks Arch Surg. 2010;395(8):1025-30.
14. Jafari MD, Lee KH, Halabi WJ, Mills SD, Carmichael JC, Stamos MJ, et al. The use of indocyanine green fluorescence to assess anastomotic perfusion during robotic assisted laparoscopic rectal surgery. Surg Endosc. 2013;27(8):3003-8.

15. Colavita PD, Wormer BA, Belyansky I, Lincourt A, Getz SB, Heniford BT, et al. Intraoperative indocyanine green fluorescence angiography to predict wound complications in complex ventral hernia repair. Hernia. 2016;20(1):139-49.
16. Hope-Ross M, Yannuzzi LA, Gragoudas ES, Guyer DR, Slakter JS, Sorenson JA, et al. Adverse reactions due to indocyanine green. Ophthalmology. 1994;101(3): 529-33.
17. Boni L, David G, Dionigi G, Rausei S, Cassinotti E, Fingerhut A. Indocyanine green-enhanced fluorescence to assess bowel perfusion during laparoscopic colorectal resection. Surg Endosc. 2016;30(7):2736-42.
18. Alander JT, Kaartinen I, Laakso A, Pätilä T, Spillmann T, Tuchin VV, et al. A Review of indocyanine green fluorescent imaging in surgery. Int J Biomed Imaging. 2012;2012:940585.
19. Liu Z, Song D, Li Z, Peng X, Zhou B, Lü C, et al. Application progress of indocyanine green angiography in breast reconstruction. Zhongguo Xiu Fu Chong Jian Wai Ke Za Zhi. 2018;32(11):1463-8.
20. Gandhi J, Banker A, Chaudhari S, Shinde P. Role of Indocyanine Green to Mitigate Wound Complications in Component Separation Technique for Ventral Hernia Repair-Our Early Experience. World J Surg. 2021;45(10):3073-9.
21. Keller DS, Ishizawa T, Cohen R, Chand M. Indocyanine green fluorescence imaging in colorectal surgery: overview, applications, and future directions. Lancet Gastroenterol Hepatol. 2017;2(10):757-66.
22. Vallance A, Wexner S, Berho M, Cahill R, Coleman M, Haboubi N, et al. A collaborative review of the current concepts and challenges of anastomotic leaks in colorectal surgery. Colorectal Dis. 2017;19(1):O1-O12.
23. Mangano A, Masrur MA, Bustos R, Chen LL, Fernandes E, Giulianotti PC. Near-Infrared Indocyanine Green-Enhanced Fluorescence and Minimally Invasive Colorectal Surgery: Review of the Literature. Surg Technol Int. 2018;33:77-83.
24. Bobel MC, Altman A, Gaertner WB. Immunofluorescence in Robotic Colon and Rectal Surgery. Clin Colon Rectal Surg. 2021;34(5):338-44.
25. Carus T, Pick P. Intraoperative fluorescence angiography in colorectal surgery. Chirurg. 2019;90(11):887-90.
26. Hayami S, Matsuda K, Iwamoto H, Ueno M, Kawai M, Hirono S, et al. Visualization and quantification of anastomotic perfusion in colorectal surgery using near-infrared fluorescence. Tech Coloproctol. 2019;23(10):973-80.
27. Sherwinter DA, Gallagher J, Donkar T. Intra-operative transanal near infrared imaging of colorectal anastomotic perfusion: A feasibility study. Colorectal Dis. 2013;15(1):91-6.
28. Ris F, Hompes R, Cunningham C, Lindsey I, Guy R, Jones O, et al. Near-infrared (NIR) perfusion angiography in minimally invasive colorectal surgery. Surg Endosc. 2014;28(7):2221-6.
29. Watanabe J, Ota M, Suwa Y, Suzuki S, Suwa H, Momiyama M, et al. Evaluation of the intestinal blood flow near the rectosigmoid junction using the indocyanine green fluorescence method in a colorectal cancer surgery. Int J Colorectal Dis. 2015;30(3):329-35.
30. Degett TH, Andersen HS, Gögenur I. Indocyanine green fluorescence angiography for intraoperative assessment of gastrointestinal anastomotic perfusion: a systematic review of clinical trials. Langenbecks Arch Surg. 2016;401(6):767-75.

31. Jafari MD, Wexner SD, Martz JE, McLemore EC, Margolin DA, Sherwinter DA, et al. Perfusion assessment in laparoscopic left-sided/anterior resection (PILLAR II): a multi-institutional study. J Am Coll Surg. 2015;220(1):82-92.e1.
32. Marcelissen TAT, den Hollander PP, Tuytten TRAH, Sosef MN. Incidence of Iatrogenic Ureteral Injury During Open and Laparoscopic Colorectal Surgery: A Single Center Experience and Review of the Literature. Surg Laparosc Endosc Percutan Tech. 2016;26(6):513-5.
33. da Silva G, Boutros M, Wexner SD. Role of prophylactic ureteric stents in colorectal surgery. Asian J Endosc Surg. 2012;5(3):105-10.
34. Feingold DL, Addona T, Forde KA, Arnell TD, Carter JJ, Huang EH, et al. Safety and reliability of tattooing colorectal neoplasms prior to laparoscopic resection. J Gastrointest Surg. 2004;8(5):543-6.
35. Peltrini R, Podda M, Castiglioni S, di Nuzzo MM, D'Ambra M, Lionetti R, et al. Intraoperative use of indocyanine green fluorescence imaging in rectal cancer surgery: The state of the art. World J Gastroenterol. 2021;27(38):6374-86.
36. Currie AC, Brigic A, Thomas-Gibson S, Suzuki N, Moorghen M, Jenkins JT, et al. A pilot study to assess near infrared laparoscopy with indocyanine green (ICG) for intraoperative sentinel lymph node mapping in early colon cancer. Eur J Surg Oncol. 2017;43(11):2044-51.
37. Yeung TM, Wang LM, Colling R, Kraus R, Cahill R, Hompes R, et al. Intraoperative identification and analysis of lymph nodes at laparoscopic colorectal cancer surgery using fluorescence imaging combined with rapid OSNA pathological assessment. Surg Endosc. 2018;32(2):1073-6.
38. Cahill RA, Anderson M, Wang LM, Lindsey I, Cunningham C, Mortensen NJ. Near-infrared (NIR) laparoscopy for intraoperative lymphatic road-mapping and sentinel node identification during definitive surgical resection of early-stage colorectal neoplasia. Surg Endosc. 2012;26(1):197-204.
39. Nagata J, Fukunaga Y, Akiyoshi T, Konishi T, Fujimoto Y, Nagayama S, et al. Colonic Marking With Near-Infrared, Light-Emitting, Diode-Activated Indocyanine Green for Laparoscopic Colorectal Surgery. Dis Colon Rect. 2016;59(2):e14-8.
40. Zhou SC, Tian YT, Wang XW, Zhao CD, Ma S, Jiang J, et al. Application of indocyanine green-enhanced near-infrared fluorescence-guided imaging in laparoscopic lateral pelvic lymph node dissection for middle-low rectal cancer. World J Gastroenterol. 2019;25(31):4502-11.
41. Kazanowski M, al Furajii H, Cahill RA. Near-infrared laparoscopic fluorescence for pelvic side wall delta mapping in patients with rectal cancer—'PINPOINT' nodal assessment. Colorectal Dis. 2015;17 (Suppl 3):32-5.
42. Baltussen EJM, Kok END, Brouwer de Koning SG, Sanders J, Aalbers AGJ, Kok NFM, et al. Hyperspectral imaging for tissue classification, a way toward smart laparoscopic colorectal surgery. J Biomed Opt. 2019;24(1):1.
43. Rehman A Ul, Qureshi SA. A review of the medical hyperspectral imaging systems and unmixing algorithms' in biological tissues. Photodiagnosis Photodyn Ther. 2021;33:102165.
44. Kho E, de Boer LL, van de Vijver KK, van Duijnhoven F, Peeters MJTFDV, Sterenborg HJCM, et al. Hyperspectral imaging for resection margin assessment during cancer surgery. Clin Cancer Res. 2019;25(12):3572-80.
45. Gao L, Smith RT. Optical hyperspectral imaging in microscopy and spectroscopy—A review of data acquisition. J Biophotonics. 2015;8(6):441-56.

46. Jansen-Winkeln B, Barberio M, Chalopin C, Schierle K, Diana M, Köhler H, et al. Feedforward Artificial Neural Network-Based Colorectal Cancer Detection Using Hyperspectral Imaging: A Step towards Automatic Optical Biopsy. Cancers. 2021;13(5):1-14.
47. Akbari H, Kosugi Y, Kojima K, Tanaka N. Detection and analysis of the intestinal ischemia using visible and invisible hyperspectral imaging. IEEE Trans Biomed Eng. 2010;57(8):2011-7.
48. Kulcke A, Holmer A, Wahl P, Siemers F, Wild T, Daeschlein G. A compact hyperspectral camera for measurement of perfusion parameters in medicine. Biomedizinische Technik. 2018;63(5):547-56.
49. Jansen-Winkeln B, Holfert N, Köhler H, Moulla Y, Takoh JP, Rabe SM, et al. Determination of the transection margin during colorectal resection with hyperspectral imaging (HSI). Int J Colorectal Dis. 2019;34(4):731-9.
50. Jansen-Winkeln B, Germann I, Köhler H, Mehdorn M, Maktabi M, Sucher R, et al. Comparison of hyperspectral imaging and fluorescence angiography for the determination of the transection margin in colorectal resections-a comparative study. Int J Colorectal Dis. 2021;36(2):283-91.

Robotic Esophageal Resections: Improving Outcomes

CHAPTER 6

Kalyan Pandey

■ INTRODUCTION

When we talk about esophagectomy we presume that it is for esophageal cancer, we usually forget other indications such as Barrett's esophagitis, stricture of the esophagus, and "burned out esophagus" a sequelae of achalasia, and Chagas disease[1] nevertheless esophageal cancer is the most common indication of esophagectomy and it will not be wrong if we limit our discussion on esophagectomy for esophageal cancer only. Esophageal cancer is eighth most common cancer in the world and sixth most common cause of cancer mortality.[2] Sex distribution is equal for squamous cell carcinoma (SCC), but adenocarcinoma is three times more common in males than in females. As per World Health Organization (WHO), carcinoma esophagus is the sixth most common cancer in India, with incidence of 5.04%; it is the fifth most common cancer in males and sixth most common cancer in female. The male to female ratio is 2.4:1.[3] Risk factors for SCC are smoking and alcohol consumption; adenocarcinoma predominantly occurs in patients with gastroesophageal reflux disease or obesity.[1,4] There is paradigm shift in management of carcinoma esophagus with emergence of many center of excellence. Advances in staging, surgical technology, neoadjuvant therapy, and perioperative care have reduced morbidity and mortality.[4]

The standard treatment for patients with resectable esophageal neoplasm is esophagectomy with locoregional lymphadenectomy. Esophagectomy is technically demanding operation. In spite of medical advances, it is still associated with morbidity in 40–50% of cases, mortality in 8–11% of cases and low survival rate of 15–25% at 5 years.[4]

Franz Torek was the first to describe resection of esophagus he used a rubber tube for an extra-anatomic reconstruction.[5] Interestingly, the patient survived for 13 years. This led to the evolution of esophageal surgery. Traditionally open esophagectomy (OE) has been the surgical treatment of choice;[6] it can be transhiatal or Ivor Lewis or McKeown esophagectomy.[7,8] The choice of technique depends on several factors such as the location of the tumor, an institution's resources, and the experience of operating surgeon.[9]

Minimally invasive techniques were introduced in the early 1990s to decrease the morbidity associated with esophagectomy.[9] Multiple studies have demonstrated a decrease in perioperative complications[10] but the data describing oncologic outcomes, specifically regarding the extent of lymph node dissection, are varied.[11]

Robotic-assisted minimally invasive esophagectomy (RAMIE) is an alternative to conventional minimally invasive esophagectomy (MIE), and has been increasingly applied to the treatment of esophageal cancer.[12] The benefits include: a superior quality three-dimensional (3D) image and free articulation of the tips of the robotic instruments which assist in more precise manner, especially enhancing the lymph node dissection.[12] Increasingly studies are demonstrating that robotic esophagectomy decrease morbidity, mortality, patients report better quality of life (QOL), physical function, and less fatigue, and pain at 3 months after surgery.[13] Nonetheless, while robotic-assisted esophagectomy is promising but, technical difficulties, long operating times, and lack of experience make this procedure difficult to adopt.[14] At present, there is no convincing data on how beneficial and to what extent RAMIE resection provides superior perioperative and oncologic outcomes, increased cost-effectiveness, and improved QOL remain unclear.[15,13,14]

■ MINIMALLY INVASIVE TECHNIQUES

Esophagectomy is a complex procedure requiring thoracic, abdominal and cervical approach.[15,13] Several factors influence postoperative and long-term outcomes: patient selection, surgical procedure selection, standardized perioperative protocols, prompt intervention in the treatment of post-operative complications.[16] Equally important is the skill of operating surgical team hence surgery should be performed only in centers with minimum 20 cases per year.

Open transthoracic esophagectomy is gold standard; it allows complete tumor resection (R0), extended lymphadenectomy, and restoration of digestive tract with intrathoracic, or cervical anastomosis; intraoperative complications are also low in open surgery.[14] The systemic inflammatory response due to trauma from thoracotomy and/or laparotomy led to the introduction of minimally invasive surgical techniques in esophagectomy.[17] The first results of MIE reported in the medical literature in 1992 when the first thoracoscopic esophagectomy was performed by Sir Alfred Cuschieri.[18]

Indications for minimally-invasive esophagectomy are similar to those for OE. The relative contraindications are known extensive pleural or abdominal adhesions, the absolute contraindication are the inability to use single-lung ventilation because of previous resection or poor lung function.[19,20] Surgeon expertise and experience are additional important factors.

Anastomotic techniques in MIEs have varied with surgeons. Cervical and thoracic anastomosis techniques which have been described are either handsewn, circular, or linear stapled anastomotic technique. More recently, the OrVil (Covidien, Mansfield, MA, USA), which is a stapling device, has been utilized transorally, the benefits include the elimination of the technical assistance needed to attach the anvil to the esophagus.[14] Surgeons also differ on whether or not to perform a pyloroplasty or pyloromyotomy, or Botox injection, or prophylactic thoracic duct ligation. None of above have demonstrated a substantial difference in outcomes.[14,19]

■ ROBOTIC ESOPHAGECTOMY

The use of minimally invasive techniques has many advantages including lower respiratory complications and equivalent 30-day mortality;[21] it also has many drawbacks: visualization is limited to two dimensions—(1) straight and (2) rigid instruments (limited range of motion). Instrument tips are controlled at a distance, reduced dexterity, precision, and control. Unsteady camera controlled by assistant, greater surgeon fatigue, makes complex operations more difficult. The intercostal spaces (ICSs) function as a fulcrum in thoracoscopy, it often leads to nerve injury, postoperative pain, and paresthesias.[12,22] Robotic surgery bypass these challenges using computer-assisted surgical systems.[23]

Melvin et al.[24] in 2002 reported first robotic esophagectomy, and, in 2003, Horgan described first robotic-assisted transhiatal esophagectomy (THE). Kernstine et al.[23] described the first totally robotic McKeown three-field esophagectomy in 2004. Dunn et al.[25] were the first to report the long-term outcomes of their 3-year experience of THE. There are several additional combinations of thoracic and abdominal phases of esophagectomy including video-assisted thoracoscopic surgery (VATS)/mini-thoracotomy and laparoscopy/mini-laparotomy/handport or traditional laparotomy (also known as the hybrid robotic esophagectomy).[26,27]

The use of robotics provides several advantages. Most importantly are:[12,28]

- Binocular stereoscopic 3D vision with stability of camera
- Endowrist instrumentation—increased dexterity
- High definition camera with 15x magnification
- Precise incision and dissection in tissue planes
- Extremely easy and fast intracorporeal suturing and knotting
- Surgeons sits and operates at ease with arms rested
- Multitasking instrumentations
- Option of harmonic robotic arm
- Three arms in addition to 3D HD robotic camera arm
- No tremor

- The fulcrum lies inside the body instead of resting on the body wall, which reduces postoperative pain
- Ergonomic with equal access with both left- and right-sided ports

There are some important disadvantages also:
- Access to robotic platforms
- The expense attached to their use
- Need to justify the cost associated with the procedure
- Unfamiliarity of this platform in the aging surgeon population
- Lack of training in new graduates
- Lack of trained technical and supporting staff[12]

LEARNING CURVE OF MINIMALLY INVASIVE AND ROBOTIC ESOPHAGECTOMY

Laparoscopic or robotic-assisted procedures are technically complex and have significant learning curves. Decker et al.[29] based on their study concluded that centers performing 50 or more cases had lower morbidity and mortality rates, better lymph node dissection than centers with less expertise. Around 35–40 operations are needed to attain proficiency, with 25 cases used as a benchmark for competent lymphadenectomy.[30]

The reports are somewhat varied for robotic esophagectomy, Park et al.[30] in their retrospective study found that it needed 20 cases to attain proficiency. Zhang et al.[31] concluded that 26 cases were required to gain proficiency of robotic-assisted McKeown esophagectomy. The learning curve for esophageal dissection was 26 cases and stomach mobilization requires 14 cases.[31] The bedside assistant at least needs nine cases to achieve an optimal thoracic docking, and 16 cases for abdominal docking and assistance.[31] When we compare minimally invasive surgery (MIS) to robotic esophagectomy we find that the learning curve is less in robotic as shown in **Figure 1**.

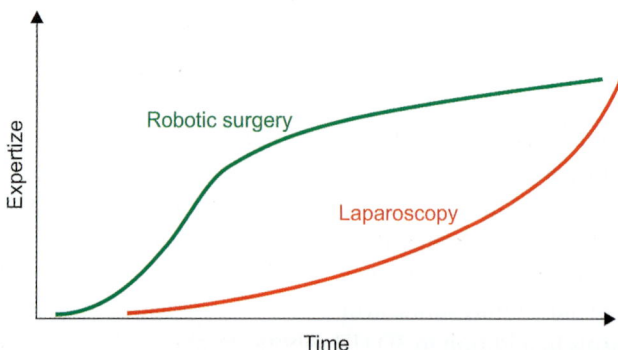

Fig. 1: Learning curve of minimally invasive surgery (MIS) and robotic esophagectomy.

In a paper published by us in Indian Journal of Surgery in 2015 with experience of 35 patients we found that the time taken for first 10 cases was comparatively longer than next 25 cases also the blood loss was lower and rate of complications was also less compared to first 10 cases.[12]

OUTCOME OF OPEN VERSUS MIS VERSUS ROBOTIC-ASSISTED ESOPHAGECTOMY

Comparison between OE to minimally invasive techniques will help to determine the benefits of MIE.[32] Naffouje et al.[33] reported their results of a propensity score-matched analysis using the National Surgical Quality Improvement Program (NSQIP) database evaluating participants who underwent OE or MIE. One 161 open transthoracic esophagectomy (OTTE) patients were matched with MIEs patients in ratio of 1:1, the OTTE subgroup had higher completion rates of abdominal and mediastinal lymph node dissection (26.7% vs. 3.1% and 38.5% vs. 16.1%, respectively; $p < 0.001$) and shorter mean operative time (329 min vs. 414 min; $p < 0.001$).[33] But, higher rates of wound complications were reported in the OTTE population (7.5% vs. 1.9%), also the median hospitalization was longer (10 days vs. 8 days), more patients required discharge to a facility (18.0% vs. 8.1%), and postoperative blood transfusion (13.0% vs. 6.8%; $p = 0.092$). They concluded that the OTTE cohort demonstrated higher complication rates (46.0% vs. 33.5%; $p = 0.028$); but no difference in attaining negative margins, anastomotic leak, need for reoperation, readmission, or mortality.[33] Robotic esophagectomy also resulted in higher mediastinal lymph node yield.[33,34]

Zhang et al.[35] more recently compared laparoscopic esophagectomy to robotic esophagectomy. study included 66 matched pairs also using propensity score-matched cohorts, they reported operative time in the robot-assisted Ivor Lewis esophagectomy (RAILE) group to be significantly longer than that in the thoracoscopic-assisted Ivor Lewis (TAIL) group (302.0 ± 62.9 min vs. 274.7 ± 38.0 min, $p = 0.004$). With no significant difference in the rates of overall complications (28.8% vs. 24.2%, $p = 0.554$), blood loss {200.0 mL [interquartile range (IQR) 100.0–262.5 mL] vs. 200.0 mL (IQR 150.0–245.0 mL), $p = 0.100$}, length of stay [9.0 days (IQR 8.0–12.3 days) vs. 9.0 days (IQR 8.0–11.3 days), $p = 0.517$], and total number of dissected lymph nodes (19.2 ± 9.2 vs. 19.3 ± 9.5, $p = 0.955$). There were two conversions in the RAILE group, and no 30-day readmissions.

If we see direct comparison of open to robotic esophagectomy, van der Sluis et al.[36] in a randomized controlled trial evaluated the robot-assisted minimally invasive thoracic and laparoscopic esophagectomy versus open transthoracic esophagectomy for resectable esophageal cancer (ROBOT trial). This was the only study which evaluated long-term (5 years) outcome of robotic-assisted esophagectomy. This was a single-center randomized controlled parallel-group, superiority trial and included all adult patients (age ≥18 and ≤80 years) who demonstrated a performance status in line with the European Clinical Oncology Group scoring of 0, 1, or 2, had biopsy proven, surgically resectable (cT1-4a, N0-3, M0) mid and lower esophageal cancer.[37] Primary outcome was the percentage of overall complications (grade 2 and higher) according to the modified Clavien–Dindo classification. Trial started in January 2012 and patients were followed for 5 years. In total, 112 patients who fulfilled the criteria were randomly assigned to either RAMIE or OTTE. The primary endpoint was occurrence of surgery-related postoperative complications.

The RAMIE (59%) group experienced fewer surgery-related postoperative complications compared to the OTTE (80%) group [risk ratio (RR) with RAMIE 0.74; 95% confidence interval (CI): 0.57–0.96; $p = 0.02$], less median blood loss (400 mL vs. 568 mL, $p < 0.001$), fewer pulmonary (RR: 0.54; 95% CI: 0.34–0.85; $p = 0.005$) and cardiac complications (RR: 0.47; 95% CI: 0.27–0.83; $p = 0.006$), also less postoperative pain (mean visual analog scale, 1.86 vs. 2.62; $p < 0.001$) compared to OTTE.[38] Participants reported better functional recovery in the RAMIE population by POD 14, (RR: 1.48, 95% CI: 1.03–2.13; $p = 0.038$) and the QOL score was better at discharge [mean difference QOL score 13.4 (2.0–24.7, $p = 0.02$)] and 6 weeks thereafter [mean difference 11.1 QOL score (1.0–21.1; $p = 0.03$)]. Most importantly, oncologic outcomes were comparable in both short- and long-term at a medium follow-up (40 months).[36]

It is also important to mention the cost differences among the open, minimally invasive, and robotic techniques. Proponents of minimally invasive and robotic techniques have stated that, although MIS incur a higher surgical expenditure, it is counterbalanced by the savings through an accelerated recovery. Conversely, critics suggest that the added cost of MIE and robotic procedures is often not recovered in the postoperative period, despite the decreased or lack of intensive care unit (ICU) stay. Lee et al.[39] with help of a decision-analysis model compared the estimated costs of MIE to OE and found that, MIE cost less than OE, over a 1-year time period. Others found similar findings of lower overall cost at different time points, which were also attributed to decreased postoperative costs.[38] Conversely, Liu et al.[40] compared MIE to OE and found that, even though the postoperative costs of MIE were significantly lower, this did not offset the higher procedural expense.[41]

■ HOW WE DO IT? THE MANIPAL EXPERIENCE

Preoperative Evaluation

Apart from clinical and endoscopic examination, a computerized tomography (thoracic and abdominal) for the evaluation of the tumor and to rule out metastases. We routinely use positron emission tomography-computed tomography (PET-CT) in all the cases for staging, as it can avoid unnecessary surgery. However, PET has limitations, peritumoral lymph nodes are often difficult to assess due to the proximity of the primary tumor. Endoscopic ultrasound is used for assessment of the local lymph node when the tumor is not completely stenotic. A bronchoscopy is recommended for tumors located above the carina or those in close contact with the left bronchus to look for recurrent laryngeal nerve involvement and tracheal infiltration. Diagnostic laparoscopy is done to exclude peritoneal metastases; in locally advanced distal esophageal adenocarcinoma (T3/T4), peritoneal metastasis is 15% of such patients. Pulmonary function test and cardiological evaluation are mandatory. The prognosis of patients is determined by tumor stage, histological type, differentiation, and the location of the tumor.

Multimodal therapy has improved the overall survival, it can be chemotherapy or a combination of chemotherapy and radiation based of tumor type location and institutional preference. In patients in early stages of disease (cT1-2N0), upfront esophagectomy is recommended. Neoadjuvant therapy is indicated in stage IIb-III, because it increases resectability rate and survival, surgery is rarely an option for stage IV patients and only complements palliative treatment. At our institute we usually subject the patient to neoadjuvant chemotherapy (NACT) with TPF regimen, FLOT, or FOLFOX are acceptable alternatives based on discretion of medical oncologist and multidisciplinary board which we recommend for all oncology centers.

During neoadjuvant therapy nutrition is paramount and patient may need nasogastric tube insertion or feeding jejunostomy. We do not prefer gastrostomy to avoid compromising future reconstruction options. Malnutrition is associated with increased operative risk and is associated with low survival.

Preoperative Assessment and Preparation

Preoperative investigations needed for surgery and anesthesia purpose are complete blood count, coagulation, and hepatic and renal function are assessed, electrocardiogram, 2D Echo, chest X-ray, and pulmonary function tests.

We follow enhanced recovery after surgery (ERAS) protocol in our institute. Patients take clear liquids with oral antibiotics one day prior to surgery, are kept fasting for 6 hours, also carbo-load with 150 mg of glucose is given 2 hours before surgery to nondiabetic patients. Low molecular weight heparin is started on the day of surgery till the patient is mobilized.

Operative System

We use Da Vinci X system at our institute. We are privileged to have a dedicated robotic theater and operating team which makes our life easy.

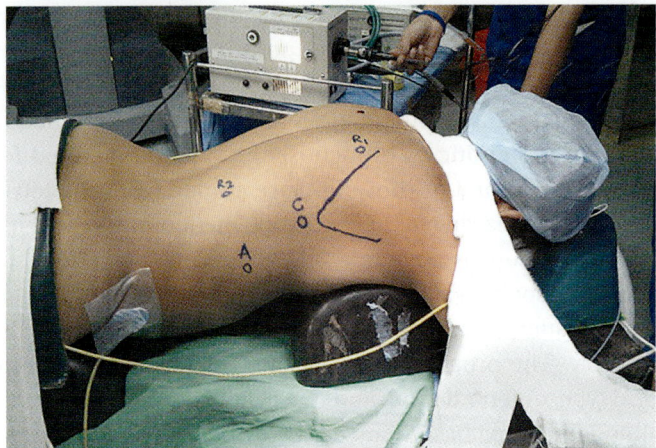

Fig. 2: Patient positioning and port markings.

Anesthesia and Patient Positioning

After induction of general anesthesia and intubation with double lumen tube, placement of central line, arterial line, nasogastric tube, and Foley catheter is done. Paravertebral intercostal block in 6 ICS is used for all cases for pain management. We use prone position for thoracic part of procedure thus patient is turned prone on sandbag and single lung ventilation is started **(Fig. 2)**.

Tips and Trick
- All had paravertebral intercostal block
- *Little underhydration peroperative:* Changing mindset of anesthetists!!!
- To accept little low urine output intraoperatively
- Extubate all patients postoperatively

Operation Technique

We perform total robotic esophagectomy (robotic-assisted transthoracic and transperitoneal three-stage esophagectomy) which is done in three phases:
1. Thoracic phase
2. Abdominal phase
3. Cervical phase

Thoracic Phase

At our center we use three robotic and one assistant port for thoracic phase. The third arm of the robot is not used. Placement of ports is shown in **Figure 3**; camera port is inserted one finger breadth below the tip of scapula usually in 7th intercostal spaces, two additional 8 mm ports are

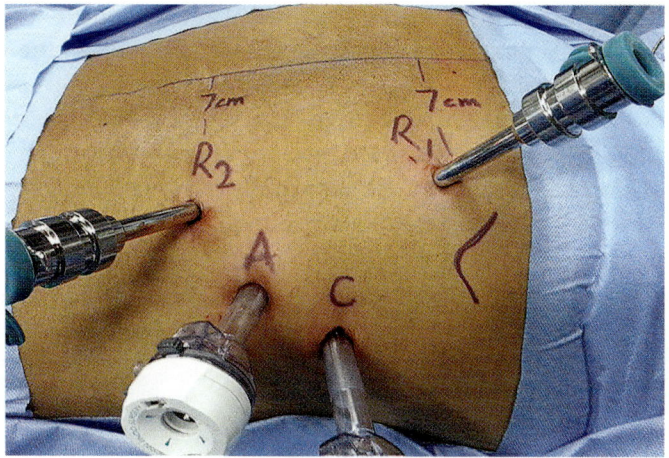

Fig. 3: Port placement after painting and draping.

inserted under direct vision in a vertical line 5 cm apart and in triangulation with camera port at a minimum distance of 7 cm from midline. One 10 mm assistant port is placed between left working port and camera port; this is used for suctioning and clip application, CO_2 gas insufflation is done to maintain a pressure of 10 mm Hg.

We use bipolar forceps in left arm and hot shears in right arm, the procedure begins with incision of the visceral pleura between esophagus and lung just inferior to the azygos vein, this helps in keeping esophagus attached to the pleura on aortic side, more than three-fourths of esophagus is mobilized in this way from the cranial to caudal direction taking down inferior pulmonary ligament and up to hiatus caudally, the direct large aortic branches are clipped and smaller ones are bipolarized, an umbilical tape looped around esophagus helps in traction. Vagal fibers going to bronchus are preserved and distal branches are divided. Azygos vein is clipped and divided and the same dissection is continued in the supra-azygos region **(Figs. 4 and 5)**.

During supra-azygos dissection, it is paramount to preserve recurrent laryngeal nerve. It is to be noted that one must remove lower and middle mediastinal, subcarinal, and right paratracheal nodes along with specimen. After completion of thoracic part two 24F drains are placed one anteriorly toward the apex and other one posteriorly toward the base **(Figs. 6A to D)**.

The advantages of prone position during the thoracoscopic esophagectomy are: (1) better exposure of the intrathoracic anatomical structures without fully collapsing the right lung which can reduce the postoperative respiratory complications. (2) A better approach is obtained at the level of the right hemithorax compared to the standard left lateral position, (3) less amplitude of movement of the mediastinum, (4) the exposure is superior behind the right pulmonary hill with easier visualization of the vascular elements, (5) the lung is moved away from the operative field of esophageal dissection by its own weight, and (6) the esophagus is the highest point of right hemithorax, and thus the blood resulting from the dissection does not obscure the operative field (as opposed to the left lateral left decubitus in which the blood stagnates in the dissection area).

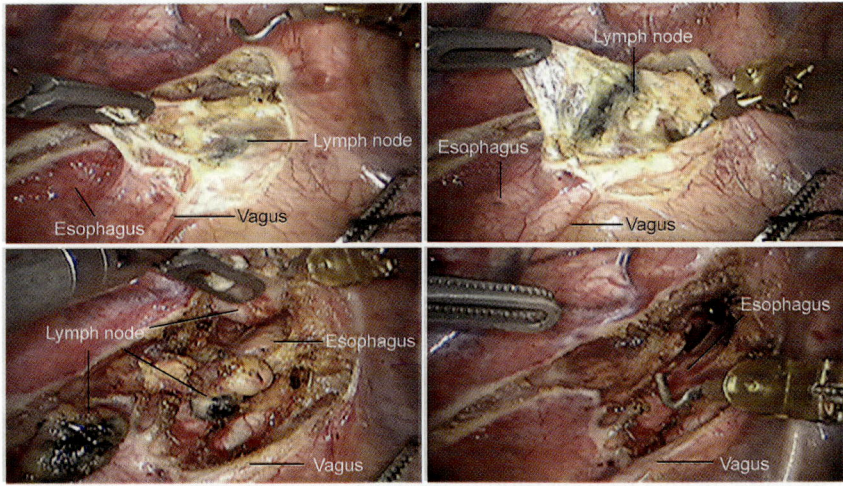

Fig. 4: Operative steps of thoracic esophagectomy.

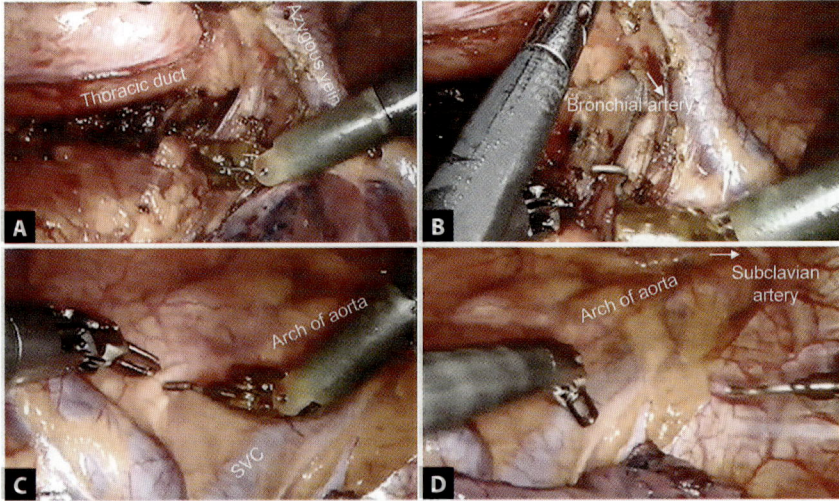

Figs. 5A to B: Intrathoracic dissection demonstrating: (A) Thoracic duct; (B) Right bronchial artery; (C) Superior vena cava (SVC) and arch of aorta; (D) Right subclavian artery.

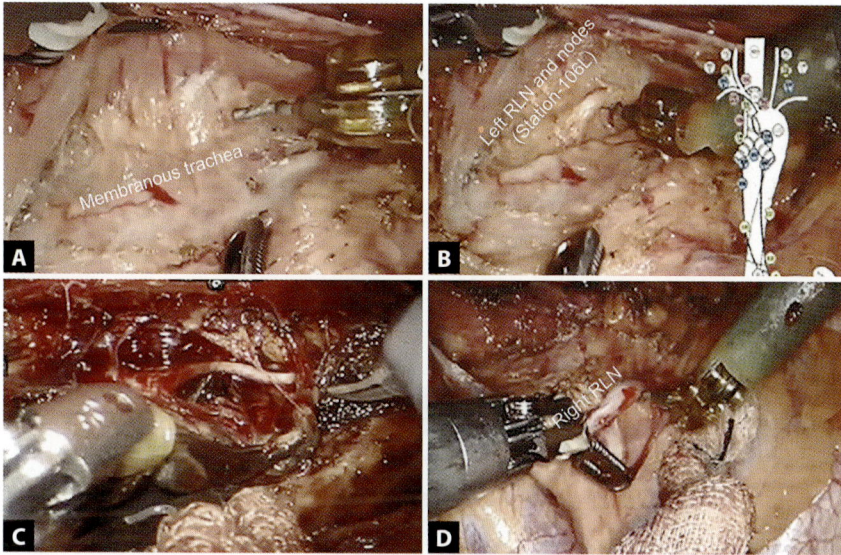

Figs. 6A to D: Intrathoracic supra-azygos dissection demonstrating: (A) Membranous part of trachea; (B and C) Left recurrent laryngeal nerve (RLN) and nodal dissection around it; (D) Right RLN.

Abdominal Phase

After esophageal phase, the patient is repositioned to supine with neck extension which helps in cervical phase and double lumen tube is replaced with single lumen tube. Ports are placed as shown in **Figure 7B**. Camera port is inserted one finger breath below the umbilicus, additional ports are placed one in right subcostal region in anterior axillary line, between camera port and right port in transpyloric plane. Another port is placed in left subcostal region in anterior axillary line. Assistant port is placed between camera port and left port with triangular fashion. We use hot shears in left port vessel sealer in R2 and bipolar in R1. Robot is redocked from head end **(Figs. 7A to D)**. Versa band is used to retract the liver. Dissection starts with division of lesser omentum, above right gastric artery till hiatus next right crus of diaphragm is divided to widen the hiatus. Care should be taken if accessory left hepatic artery is present which should be preserved if sizable **(Figs. 8A to D)**. Next is posterior dissection along superior border of pancreas till splenic hilum, during this step left gastric artery and vein are identified clipped and divided, lymph nodes along the left gastric vessels are removed along the specimen. During this step, complete D2 lymph node dissection is done by removing lymph nodes along hepatic artery, splenic vessels, and splenic hilum. The third step is division of omentum along the greater curvature; dissection is started along greater curvature, omentum is divided from pylorus to crus of diaphragm; it is utmost important to

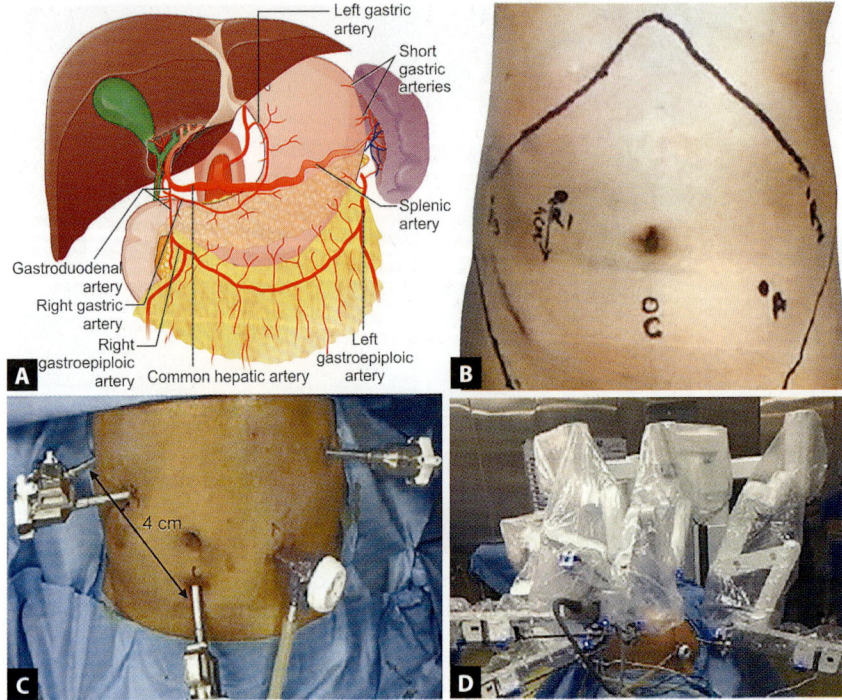

Figs. 7A to D: (A) Anatomy demonstrating structures at the level of transpyloric plane; (B and C) Surface marking and placement of abdominal ports; (D) Docking of robot from head end of patient.

preserve right gastroepiploic artery and vein which is the future supply of gastric conduit, finally thoracic and abdominal dissection are connected and adhesions at hiatus are released. Once the dissection is complete robot is undocked and mobilization of cervical esophagus is done by left supraclavicular incision.

Cervical Phase

Left supraclavicular incision of around 3–5 cm taken along the anterior border of left sternocleidomastoid muscle. Esophagus is identified and looped and mobilized recurrent laryngeal nerve is identified and preserved. Esophagus is divided and Ryles tube is tied to cut end.

Next laparotomy is done with small supraumbilical incision around 5 cm in length and wound protector is inserted. Mobilized stomach and esophagus are then delivered out, next gastric tube is made **(Fig. 9)** and pyloroplasty is done. Indocyanine green (ICG) dye is injected and vascularity is checked **(Fig. 10)**. Gastric tube is tied to Ryles tube and is pulled to the neck through cervical incision. Cervical anastomosis is done with NTLC stapler and neck wound is closed. We generally do not use abdominal and neck drains.

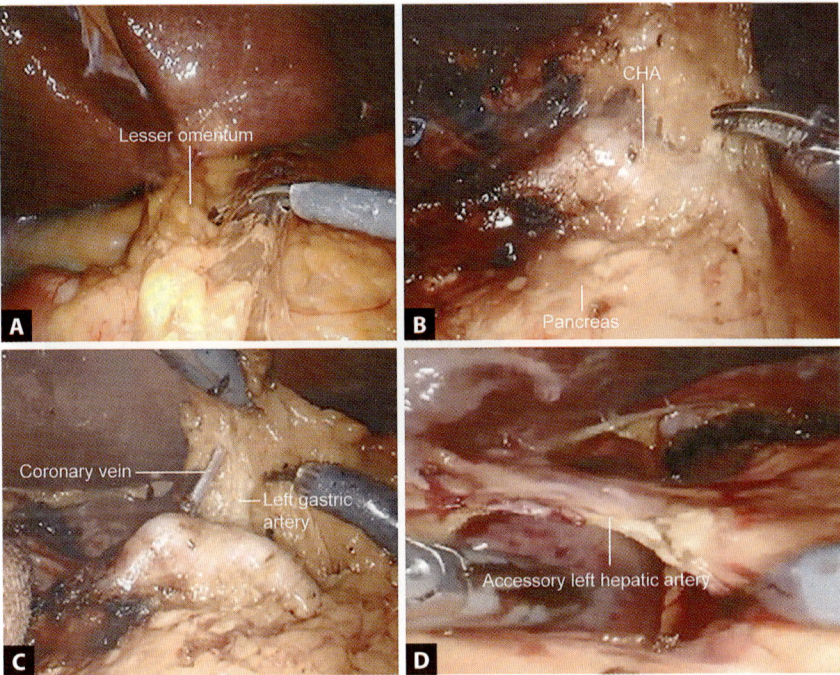

Figs. 8A to D: Intra-abdominal dissection demonstrating: (A) Lesser omentum; (B) Superior border of pancreas and common hepatic artery (CHA); (C) Left gastric artery and vein; (D) Accessory left hepatic artery.

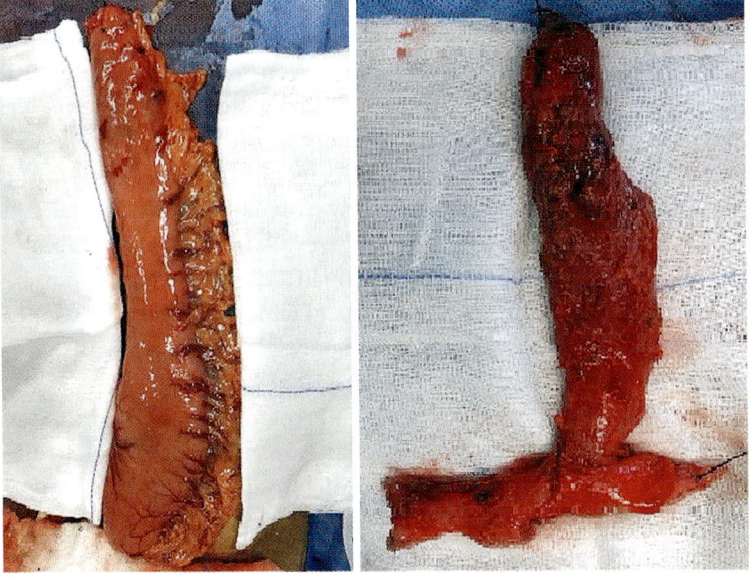

Fig. 9: Gastric conduit and specimen of esophagectomy with gastroesophageal (GE) junction and lesser curvature.

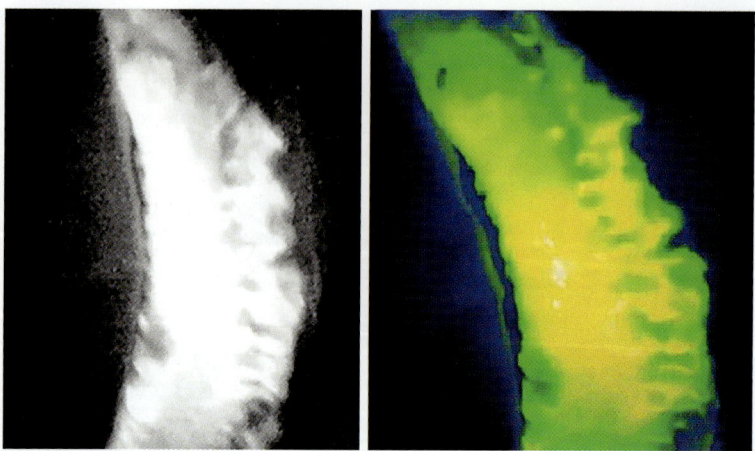

Fig. 10: Gastric conduit vascularity after indocyanine green (ICG) injection and firefly technology.

Feeding jejunostomy is done in all cases which helps in early enteral feeding and saves us (in case of) any untoward complications.

ROBOTIC ESOPHAGECTOMY DATA FROM MANIPAL HOSPITAL, BANGALORE

From November, 2011 to November, 2020 we performed 168 total robotic esophagectomies (robotic-assisted transthoracic and transperitoneal three-stage esophagectomy). We aimed to evaluate the safety and technical feasibility of total robot-assisted three-stage esophagectomy. In this period, we operated 101 male patients and 67 female patients. Median age was 61 years (range 38–72) but majority of patients were in the age group of 60–70 years. Sixty percent of the patients had associated comorbid conditions such as diabetes, hypertension, ischemic heart disease, and other illness. Histologically proven SCC or adenocarcinoma of the intrathoracic esophagus which were surgically resectable (T1-3, N0-1, M0) and could tolerate resection (ECOG performance status: 0, 1, or 2) were included in the study whereas carcinoma of cervical esophagus, patients unfit for general anesthesia and patients with stage IV disease were excluded **(Table 1)**.

Neoadjuvant chemotherapy with TPF regimen was used in stage III whereas stage I and stage II esophageal cancers were operated directly. Having said most of the patients present in advanced stage and NACT is a norm and primary surgery is an exception in our setup. Post-NACT, a partial response rate of 58.8% was achieved and 17.6% patients achieved a complete response. Technique and feasibility of robot-assisted surgery in terms of operating time, estimated blood loss, total number of lymph nodes retrieved, postoperative ventilator support, ICU stay, hospital stay, conversion to open procedure, margin status (mucosal and circumferential), and intraoperative and postoperative complications were analyzed. Complications were classified according to modified Clavien-Dindo classification of surgical complications.

Results: Total docking time for initial 10 cases was 67.90 ± 13.24 minutes, while for subsequent cases it was 33.20 ± 4.16 minutes, similarly total operative time was 429.20 ± 57.65 minutes and 321.13 ± 13.75 minutes for initial 10 cases and subsequent cases, thoracic-phase operative time for initial 10 cases and subsequent cases was 96.60 ± 20.33 minutes and 57.04 ± 9.15 minutes showing the steeper learning curve in robotics which is in contrast to minimal access surgery **(Fig. 11 and Table 2)**.

TABLE 1: Clinical profile of the patient.

Age (years)	Range 38–72
	Median 61
Sex distribution	Male: 101 (60.11%)
	Female: 67 (39.88%)
Location of tumor	Upper: 14 (8.3%)
	Middle: 75 (44.6%)
	Lower: 79 (47%)
Histology	Squamous cell carcinoma (SCC): 88 (52.38%)
	Adenocarcinoma: 80 (47.61%)

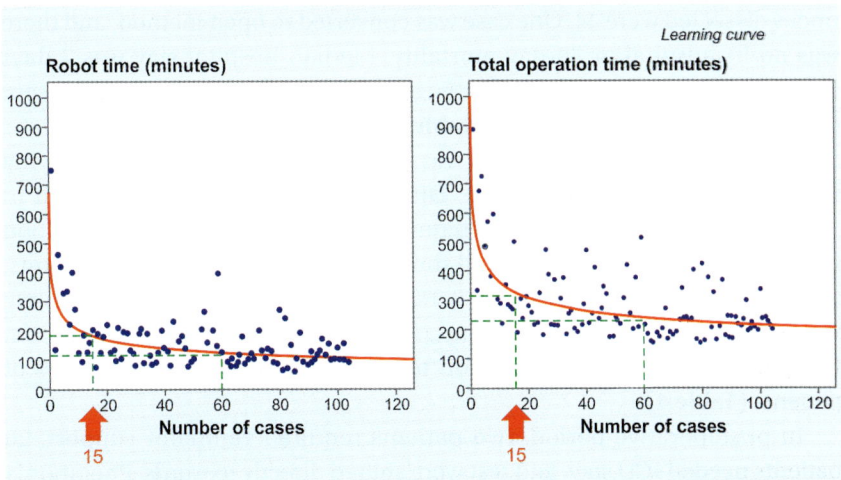

Fig. 11: Relationship between robot using time and total operating time with number of cases.

TABLE 2: Docking time and operation time.

Variables	Initial 10 cases (mean ± SD)	Subsequent cases (mean ± SD)
Total docking time (min)	67.90 ± 13.24	33.20 ± 4.16
Thoracic phase docking time (min)	32.20 ± 9.74	13.76 ± 3.43
Total operative time (thoracic, abdominal, and cervical)	429.20 ± 57.65	321.13 ± 13.75
Thoracic phase operative time (min)	96.60 ± 20.33	57.04 ± 9.15

TABLE 3: Total robotic (thoracic + abdominal esophagectomy + two-field lymphadenectomy) experience data.

Key statistics	
Lymph nodes (two-field systemic)	44
Length of stay	7 days
Vocal cord palsy	4.8%
Delayed gastric emptying	3.2%
Diaphragmatic hiatus hernia	1.6%
Reoperation	1.4%
R0 resection including CRM	98.1%
Blood loss	280.32 ± 17.52 mL

(CRM: circumferential resection margin)

The average blood loss was 280.32 ± 17.52 mL. Median numbers of lymph nodes dissected were 44. One case was converted to open method, and there was no in-hospital or 30-day mortality. Median hospital stay was 7 days (range 6–13). All had microscopic negative resection margins status except one, who had R-1 status of CRM **(Table 3)**.

Incidence of vocal cord palsy was 4.8% while delayed gastric emptying was noted in 3.2% of population. Diaphragmatic hernia was reported in 1.6% of patients, reoperation was required in 1.4% of patients average blood loss was 256 mL. We encountered thoracic duct injury in 1.6% of patients, azygos vein bleeding occurred in 0.9% of cases, pulmonary artery bleeding was encountered in 0.4% of patients, and 2% of patients suffered recurrent laryngeal nerve injury. Conversion to open surgery was done in 0.6% of patients **(Table 4)**.

In postoperative period, two patients required ventilator support, 20 patients needed ICU stay, and rest were shifted directly to wards. Pneumonia was reported in 1% of patients while pleural effusion was recorded in 2.4% of patients which required antibiotics and supportive care. We encountered

TABLE 4: Intraoperative complications (total number of patients: 168).

Complications	N = 168
Azygos vein bleeding	0.9%
Thoracic duct injury	1.6%
Pulmonary artery bleeding	0.4%
Recurrent laryngeal nerve (RLN) injury	2%
Conversion to open	0.6%

TABLE 5: Postoperative complications.

Postoperative complications	No (percentage)
Anastomotic leak	5 (2.9%)
Anastomotic stenosis	1 (0.5%)
Pulmonary embolism	0%
Deep vein thrombosis (DVT)	0%
Pneumonia	2 (1.1%)
Pleural effusion	4 (2.4%)
Permanent vocal cord palsy	1 (0.5%)
Diaphragmatic hiatal hernia	3 (1.6%)
Wound infection	1 (0.6%)
Delayed gastric emptying	6 (3.5%)
Reoperation	3 (1.7%)
60 days operative mortality	1 (0.6)%

anastomotic leak in 2.8% of patients which was managed conservatively, while anastomotic stenosis was observed in 0.5% of patients which required endoscopic dilation. The incidence of permanent vocal cord palsy was 0.6%. Sixty day operative mortality was noted in 0.59% of patients. With the longest follow-up of 50 months, 3-year disease-free survival (DFS) and overall survival (OS) were 75.4% and 68%, respectively **(Table 5)**.

■ DISCUSSION

From an open procedure involving thoracotomy and laparotomy to hybrid minimally invasive techniques, to completely minimally invasive and robotic-assisted/totally robotic techniques, surgical treatment of esophageal cancer has evolved a lot.[21] Although the advantages of minimally invasive techniques and the learning curve needed for implementation of minimally invasive esophageal surgery are still completely not clear, robotic esophagectomies have consistently demonstrated lower overall complications rates, improved scores in factors related to patient satisfaction, steeper learning curve, and robust oncologic outcomes.[32] Robotic esophagectomy results in less surgery-related and cardiopulmonary complications, lower postoperative pain, faster recovery, and improved short-term QOL in the postoperative period compared to OTTE.[42] The oncological outcomes are comparable with current standards.[12,33] Until the ROBOT trial,[36] no study had surveyed long-term outcomes or QOL metrics.

At our institute we perform robotic esophagectomy since past 10 years and we hardly do thoracotomy for esophagus since (1) we find robotic surgery much beneficial for the patient with not much cost difference; (2) the morbidity is far less as comparable to open thoracotomy, the patient is up and walking on next day of surgery and easily performs breathing exercises, the risk of pneumonia and other complications is far less than open surgery; (3) the duration of surgery is comparable to open surgery; and (4) it is precise, safe with hardly any conversion due to intraoperative complications.

Figure 12 shows the effect of number of cases on docking and operating time published by us in a study on 35 patients[12] and shows the learning curve is steeper in robotic surgery.

The average length of stay in our study is 7 days compared to 14 days in robotic and 16 days in open surgery, in a study by van der Sluis et al., the mean operative time was 296 minutes in our study compared to 340 minutes in robotic and 349 minutes in open surgery, estimated blood loss was 280 mL versus 400 mL in robotic and 569 mL in open surgery, our lymph node

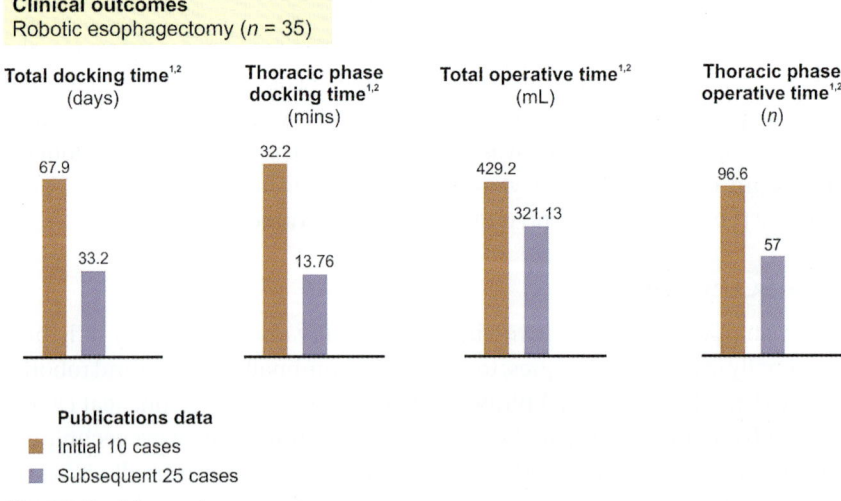

Fig. 12: Docking and surgery time.
[1]Dr Somashekar et al.: Total (transthoracic and transabdominal robotic radical three stage esophagectomy-intial indian experience.

harvest was higher as compared to harvested by them in robotic and open surgery 44 versus 27 versus 25 also 60-day mortality was only 0.6% compared to 6% in robotic and 2% in open surgery performed by them.

We encountered less intraoperative 5.5% versus 13 robotic versus 16% open and postoperative complications 18.4% versus 59% robotic versus 80% open compared to results published van der Sluis et al.,[36,37] also our reoperation rate was 1.4% versus 24% in robotic versus 33% in open surgery. R0 resection was comparable between our study 98% versus 96% in open and 93 in robotic esophagectomy performed by them. Also wound infection was comparable between robotic surgeries 0.6% versus 4% and significantly less compared to 14% in open surgery performed by them. Our conversion rate was 0.6%. Anastomotic leak was 2.8% compared to 24% in robotic surgery and 20% in open surgery performed by them. The incidence of recurrent laryngeal nerve palsy was 2% compared to 9% in robotic and 11% in open surgery performed by them. We did not encounter any incidence of pulmonary embolism compared to 6% in robotic and 2% in open surgery by van der Sluis et al.,[36,37] also the incidence of pneumonia was 1% compared to 28% and 55% in robotic and open surgery by them **(Figs. 13 to 15)**.

The limiting factors for utility of the robotic platform are the expense of robotic system and surgeon experience. While surgeons believe the needed learning curve of robotic surgery is prohibitive to its incorporation in surgical practice, interestingly van der Sluis et al.[36,37] and our study reported a much

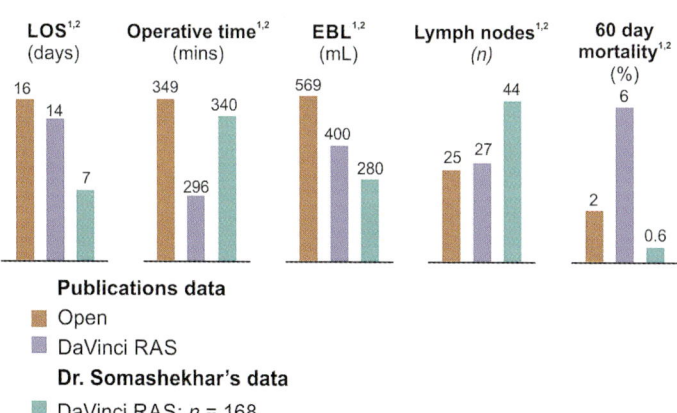

Fig. 13: Key variables comparison with van der Sluis et al.[36,37]
[1]Dr Somashekar's Robotic esophagectomy data (RAS n = 168).
[2]Van der Sluis, et al.: Robot-assisted minimally invasive thoracolaparoscopic esophagectomy versus open transthoracic esophagectomy for resectable esophageal cancer. Annals of surgery, 2018 (open N = 55, RAS N = 54).

Clinical outcomes
Robotic esophagectomy (n = 168)
Dr. Somashekhar's Robotic Esophagectomy data[1] vs. Published data (van der Sluis et al.[2])

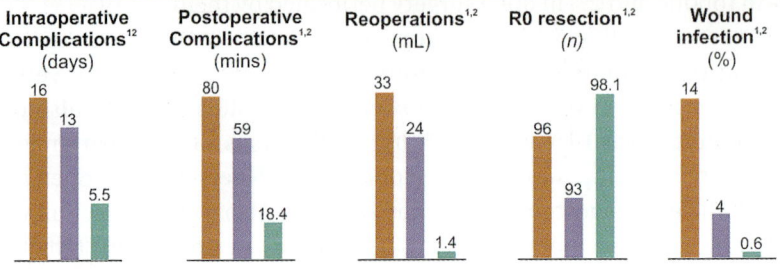

Fig. 14: Key variables comparison with van der Sluis et al.[36,37]

[1]Dr Somashekar's Robotic esophagectomy data (RAS n = 168).
[2]Van der Sluis, et al.: Robot-assisted minimally invasive thoracolaparoscopic esophagectomy versus open transthoracic esophagectomy for resectable esophageal cancer. Annals of surgery, 2018 (open N = 55, RAS N = 54).

Clinical outcomes
Robotic esophagectomy (n = 168)
Dr. Somashekhar's Robotic Esophagectomy data[1] vs. Published data (van der Sluis et al.[2])

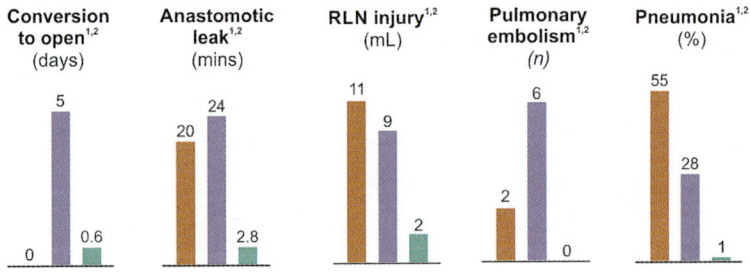

Fig. 15: Key variables comparison with van der Sluis et al.[36,37]

[1]Dr Somashekar's Robotic esophagectomy data (RAS n = 168).
[2]Van der Sluis, et al.: Robot-assisted minimally invasive thoracolaparoscopic esophagectomy versus open transthoracic esophagectomy for resectable esophageal cancer. Annals of surgery, 2018 (open N = 55, RAS N = 54).

steeper learning curve for the robotic surgery compared to the traditional MIE. Experts agree that the experience with robotic surgery and the surgeon's willingness to practice simulation are the most important factors in reducing working time to robotic competency.

Finally, we will like to highlight the limitations of this review. First, esophagectomy is a rare procedure except in few high-volume centers. The sample size is often quite small. When we compare institutional experience of MIE versus robotic procedures, MIE has a vast experience of thousands of cases with excellent outcomes. The number of robotic procedures is quite low. While MIE has proven records in regards to oncologic outcomes, and lower morbidity, robotic surgery still needs to duplicate results of MIS esophagectomy. Second, there are various types of esophagectomy that a surgeon can perform depending on experience with open, laparoscopic, thoracoscopic, and robotic techniques. Furthermore same procedure is performed in different way by different surgeon, making the comparison difficult. The perioperative pathways also differ significantly in different institutions, leading to difficult comparison. Third, Ivor Lewis esophagectomy is the most commonly performed procedure; hence most outcome data are based on comparison of this procedure type alone. Fourth, description of the specific robotic platform used in the reporting of operating times for the robotic studies has been mostly absent. Lastly, the QOL metrics has been absent from almost all studies with exception of one study,[43] the ROBOT trial. Ultimately, patient can use this information including complication rates and oncologic outcomes to make educated decisions.

■ FUTURE DIRECTIONS

Clearly there is a trend toward adoption of MIS in esophageal resections. As surgeons' MIS skills improve, surgical choices will move to either completely minimally invasive or fully robotic techniques. Additionally, as the technology will improve, surgery will become more easy. The introduction of single port[44] or robotic surgical devices has expanded the options available to achieve improved dissection and, ultimately, better oncologic outcomes.[45] Surgeons will continue to evolve and perform esophagectomy in a much safer way with ongoing improvements in robotic techniques. As the cost of robotic surgery is decreasing and the number of robotic platforms is increasing more and more patients will get the benefits of minimally invasive robotic esophagectomy **(Fig. 16)**.

■ CONCLUSION

There is a trend toward minimally invasive techniques, and robotic-assisted esophagectomy driven by the decreased morbidity and mortality of the

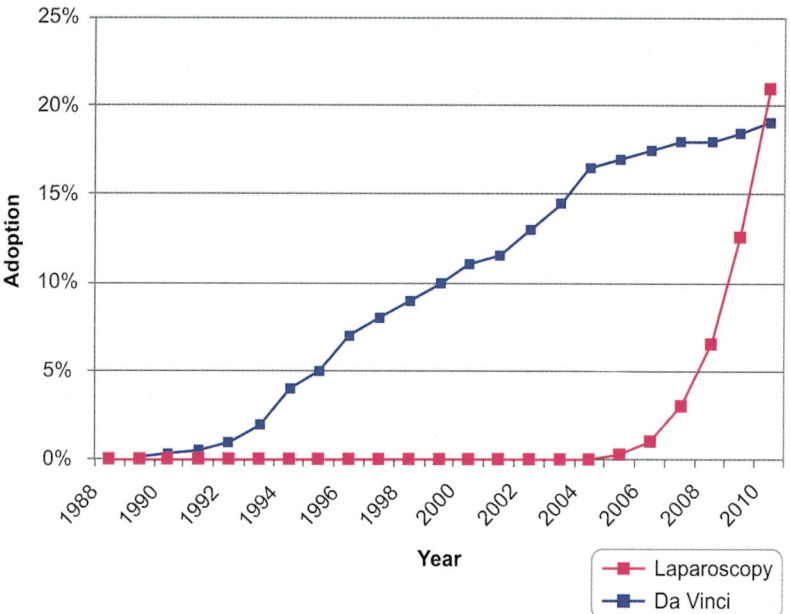

Fig. 16: Adoption of minimally invasive surgery (MIS) and Da Vinci system.

procedure. Robotic-assisted esophagectomy is the newest innovation and has benefits like an advantage of total thoracic and abdominal MIS with very low conversion rates, short learning curve, excellent chance of good quality lymphadenectomy in supra-azygos and bilateral recurrent laryngeal nerve area option for both robotic stapler and handsewn intracorporeal anastomosis. There are challenges also; notably, the need for specific teaching programs and proctored learning. As more studies confirm the lower incidence of major complications, and comparable overall and DFS compared to open approaches, the use of robotic platform to perform esophagectomy will become more common to deliver efficient oncologic care in the least invasive fashion.

■ REFERENCES

1. Malhotra GK, Yanala U, Ravipati A, Follet M, Vijayakumar M, Are C. Global trends in esophageal cancer. J Surg Oncol. 2017;115(5):564-79.
2. Mariette C, Markar SR, Dabakuyo-Yonli TS, Meunier B, Pezet D, Collet D, et al. Hybrid minimally invasive esophagectomy for esophageal cancer. N Engl J Med. 2019;380(2):152-62.
3. Indian Council of Medical Research. (2017). Consensus Document for Management of Esophageal Cancer. Available from: https://main.icmr.nic.in/sites/default/files/guidelines/Esophagus%20final%20ICMR2014_0.pdf [Last accessed December, 2022].

4. Glatz T, Marjanovic G, Kulemann B, Sick O, Hopt UT, Hoeppner J. Hybrid minimally invasive esophagectomy vs. open esophagectomy: a matched case analysis in 120 patients. Langenbecks Arch Surg. 2017;402(2):323-31.
5. Torek F. The operative treatment of carcinoma of the oesophagus. Ann Surg. 19150;61(4):385-405.
6. Lewis I. The surgical treatment of carcinoma of the oesophagus; with special reference to a new operation for growths of the middle third. Br J Surg. 1946;34:18-31.
7. McKeown KC. Total three-stage oesophagectomy for cancer of the oesophagus. Br J Surg. 1976;63(4):259-62.
8. Orringer MB, Sloan H. Esophagectomy without thoracotomy. J Thorac Cardiovasc Surg. 1978;76(5):643-54.
9. Taurchini M, Cuttitta A. Minimally invasive and robotic esophagectomy: state of the art. J Vis Surg. 2017;3:125.
10. Schumer E, Perry K, Melvin WS. Minimally invasive esophagectomy for esophageal cancer: evolution and review. Surg Laparosc Endosc Percutan Tech. 2012;22(5):383-6.
11. DePaula AL, Hashiba K, Ferreira EA, de Paula RA, Grecco E. Laparoscopic transhiatal esophagectomy with esophagogastroplasty. Surg Laparosc Endosc. 1995;5(1):1-5.
12. Somashekhar SP, Jaka RC. Total (Transthoracic and Transabdominal) Robotic Radical Three-Stage Esophagectomy-Initial Indian Experience. Indian J Surg. 2017;79(5):412-7.
13. Kauppila JH, Xie S, Johar A, Markar SR, Lagergren P. Meta-analysis of health-related quality of life after minimally invasive versus open oesophagectomy for oesophageal cancer. Br J Surg. 2017;104(9):1131-40.
14. Murthy RA, Clarke NS, Kernstine KH Sr. Minimally Invasive and Robotic Esophagectomy: A Review. Innovations (Phila). 2018;13(6):391-403.
15. Hasson RM, Fay KA, Phillips JD, Millington TM, Finley DJ. Robotic esophagectomy: the evolution of open esophagectomy to current techniques and a review of the literature. Mini-invasive Surg. 2020;4:46.
16. Torek F. The causes of failure in the operative treatment of carcinoma of the oesophagus. Ann Surg. 1929;90(4):496-506.
17. Biere SS, van Berge Henegouwen MI, Maas KW, Bonavina L, Rosman C, Garcia JR, et al. Minimally invasive versus open oesophagectomy for patients with oesophageal cancer: a multicentre, open-label, randomised controlled trial. Lancet. 2012;379(9829):1887-92.
18. Cuschieri A, Shimi S, Banting S. Endoscopic oesophagectomy through a right thoracoscopic approach. J R Coll Surg Edinb. 1992;37(1):7-11.
19. Levy RM, Trivedi D, Luketich JD. Minimally invasive esophagectomy. Surg Clin North Am. 2012;92(5):1265-85.
20. Luketich JD, Pennathur A, Awais O, Levy RM, Keeley S, Shende M, et al. Outcomes after minimally invasive esophagectomy: review of over 1000 patients. Ann Surg. 2012;256(1):95-103.
21. Suzuki Y, Urashima M, Ishibashi Y, Abo M, Omura N, Nakada K, et al. Hand-assisted laparoscopic and thoracoscopic surgery (HALTS) in radical esophagectomy with three-field lymphadenectomy for thoracic esophageal cancer. Eur J Surg Oncol. 2005;31(10):1166-74.

22. Oshikiri T, Takiguchi G, Miura S, Takase N, Hasegawa H, Yamamoto M, et al. Current status of minimally invasive esophagectomy for esophageal cancer: Is it truly less invasive? Ann Gastroenterol Surg. 2018;3(2):138-45.
23. Kernstine KH, DeArmond DT, Shamoun DM, Campos JH. The first series of completely robotic esophagectomies with three-field lymphadenectomy: initial experience. Surg Endosc. 2007;21(12):2285-92.
24. Melvin WS, Needleman BJ, Krause KR, Schneider C, Wolf RK, Michler RE, et al. Computer-enhanced robotic telesurgery. Initial experience in foregut surgery. Surg Endosc. 2002;16(12):1790-2.
25. Dunn DH, Johnson EM, Morphew JA, Dilworth HP, Krueger JL, Banerji N. Robot-assisted transhiatal esophagectomy: a 3-year single-center experience. Dis Esophagus. 2013;26(2):159-66.
26. Sarkaria IS, Rizk NP, Finley DJ, Bains MS, Adusumilli PS, Huang J, et al. Combined thoracoscopic and laparoscopic robotic-assisted minimally invasive esophagectomy using a four-arm platform: experience, technique and cautions during early procedure development. Eur J Cardiothorac Surg. 2013;43(5):e107-15.
27. Sarkaria IS, Bains MS, Finley DJ, Adusumilli PS, Huang J, Rusch VW, et al. Intraoperative near-infrared fluorescence imaging as an adjunct to robotic-assisted minimally invasive esophagectomy. Innovations (Phila). 2014;9(5):391-3.
28. Somashekhar SP, Rohit Kumar C, Rajgopal AK, Rauthan A, Patil P, Neoadjuvant chemotherapy (TPF regimen) followed with robotic surgery and its impact on outcome in management of esophageal cancers: Indian experience. J Clin Oncol. 2020;38:4_suppl:407-7.
29. Decker G, Coosemans W, De Leyn P, Decaluwé H, Nafteux P, Van Raemdonck D, et al. Minimally invasive esophagectomy for cancer. Eur J Cardiothorac Surg. 2009;35(1):13-20; discussion 20-1.
30. Park SY, Kim DJ, Kang DR, Haam SJ. Learning curve for robotic esophagectomy and dissection of bilateral recurrent laryngeal nerve nodes for esophageal cancer. Dis Esophagus. 2017;30(12):1-9.
31. Zhang H, Chen L, Wang Z, Zheng Y, Geng Y, Wang F, et al. The Learning Curve for Robotic McKeown Esophagectomy in Patients With Esophageal Cancer. Ann Thorac Surg. 2018;105(4):1024-30.
32. Patel S, Petrov R, Abbas A, Bakhos C. Robotic-assisted McKeown esophagectomy. J Vis Surg. 2019;5:43.
33. Naffouje SA, Salloum RH, Khalaf Z, Salti GI. Outcomes of Open Versus Minimally Invasive Ivor-Lewis Esophagectomy for Cancer: A Propensity-Score Matched Analysis of NSQIP Database. Ann Surg Oncol. 2019;26(7):2001-10.
34. Chao YK, Hsieh MJ, Liu YH, Liu HP. Lymph Node Evaluation in Robot-Assisted Versus Video-Assisted Thoracoscopic Esophagectomy for Esophageal Squamous Cell Carcinoma: A Propensity-Matched Analysis. World J Surg. 2018;42(2):590-8.
35. Zhang Y, Han Y, Gan Q, Xiang J, Jin R, Chen K, et al. Early Outcomes of Robot-Assisted Versus Thoracoscopic-Assisted Ivor Lewis Esophagectomy for Esophageal Cancer: A Propensity Score-Matched Study. Ann Surg Oncol. 2019;26(5):1284-91.

36. van der Sluis PC, Ruurda JP, van der Horst S, Verhage RJ, Besselink MG, Prins MJ, et al. Robot-assisted minimally invasive thoraco-laparoscopic esophagectomy versus open transthoracic esophagectomy for resectable esophageal cancer, a randomized controlled trial (ROBOT trial). Trials. 2012;13:230.
37. van der Sluis PC, van der Horst S, May AM, Schippers C, Brosens LAA, Joore HCA, et al. Robot-assisted Minimally Invasive Thoracolaparoscopic Esophagectomy Versus Open Transthoracic Esophagectomy for Resectable Esophageal Cancer: A Randomized Controlled Trial. Ann Surg. 2019;269(4):621-30.
38. Parameswaran R, Veeramootoo D, Krishnadas R, Cooper M, Berrisford R, Wajed S. Comparative experience of open and minimally invasive esophagogastric resection. World J Surg. 2009;33(9):1868-75.
39. Lee L, Sudarshan M, Li C, Latimer E, Fried GM, Mulder DS, et al. Cost-effectiveness of minimally invasive versus open esophagectomy for esophageal cancer. Ann Surg Oncol. 2013;20(12):3732-9.
40. Liu CY, Lin CS, Shih CS, Huang YA, Liu CC, Cheng CT. Cost-effectiveness of minimally invasive esophagectomy for esophageal squamous cell carcinoma. World J Surg. 2018;42(8):2522-9.
41. Dhamija A, Dhamija A, Hancock J, McCloskey B, Kim AW, Detterbeck FC, et al. Minimally invasive oesophagectomy more expensive than open despite shorter length of stay. Eur J Cardiothorac Surg. 2014;45(5):904-9.
42. Egberts JH, Schlemminger M, Hauser C, Becker T. Robot-Assisted McKeown Procedure via a Cervical Mediastinoscopy Avoiding an Abdominal and Thoracic Incision. Thorac Cardiovasc Surg. 2019;67(7):610-14.
43. Sarkaria IS, Rizk NP, Goldman DA, Sima C, Tan KS, Bains MS, et al. Early Quality of Life Outcomes After Robotic-Assisted Minimally Invasive and Open Esophagectomy. Ann Thorac Surg. 2019;108(3):920-8.
44. Fujiwara H, Shiozaki A, Konishi H, Kosuga T, Komatsu S, Ichikawa D, et al. Perioperative outcomes of single-port mediastinoscope-assisted transhiatal esophagectomy for thoracic esophageal cancer. Dis Esophagus. 2017;30(10):1-8.
45. Fujiwara H, Shiozaki A, Konishi H, Otsuji E. Transmediastinal approach for esophageal cancer: A new trend toward radical surgery. Asian J Endosc Surg. 2019;12(1):30-6.

CHAPTER 7

Perspectives on Robotic Colorectal Surgery in Today's World

Ahmed Pervez, Chelliah Selvasekar

■ INTRODUCTION

Minimal access surgery is steadily becoming the standard in the surgical management of rectal pathologies, both benign and malignant. Right at the forefront of minimal access surgery is robotic surgery. To make up for the technical shortcomings of laparoscopic surgery, the da Vinci® Surgical System was introduced by Intuitive Surgical Inc. in Sunnyvale, California, United States. The first study on robotic proctectomy was published in 2003.[1] Proponents of robotic surgery indicate several advantages, which include an enhanced three-dimensional (3D) view that eliminates hand tremors, ergonomic comfort, seven degrees of movement using microwristed instruments, and a natural hand–eye target axis.[2-4] However, despite these advantages, compared to laparoscopic surgery, the absence of an established clinical benefit and high expenses impede robotic surgery from becoming the standard of care.

In today's world, the application of robotics in colorectal surgery **(Table 1)** focuses mainly on three pathologies, namely
1. Rectal cancer
2. Rectal prolapse
3. Colon cancer.

■ ROBOTIC RECTAL CANCER SURGERY (TABLE 2)

In 2006, the first case series reporting the results of robotic anterior resection including total mesorectal excision (TME) was published **(Fig. 1)**.[5] The outcomes in robotic surgery have been evaluated as level 1B evidence[6] showing, upon comparison with laparoscopic surgery, lower or equal perioperative morbidity and hospital inpatient stay, no difference in leak rates, decreased conversion to open rates, comparable lymph node harvest, similar postoperative ileus, and no difference in R0 resection rates. Also, robotic surgery is considered valuable in some situations where laparoscopic surgery would be difficult, such as in patients with a narrow pelvis, those with a high body mass index, and male patients. Much attention is focused on autonomic nerve preservation, which gives robotic surgery an advantage

TABLE 1: Current robotic systems for colorectal surgery.

Robotic system	Features	Advantages/disadvantages
da Vinci® Xi (Intuitive surg)	Single patient cart, closed surgeon console, finger loops controllers, camera/instrument diameter of 8 mm	Multiquadrant surgery, port hopping camera, dual console, instruments can be used 10 times
Hugo™ RAS (Medtronic)	Single cart, open console with 3D glasses, a combination of finger loop and handle controllers	Portable, modular system with single/multiarmed configuration, arm hopping HD camera
CMR Surgical (Versius)	Multiple patient carts, open console with 3D glasses, joystick-like controllers, camera diameter 10 mm/instrument 5 mm	Haptic feedback, portable, independent arms, and no port docking, but the surgeon has to stand
TransEnterix (Senhance)	Multiple patient carts, open console with 3D glasses, laparoscopic handle controllers, camera/instrument diameter 3–10 mm	Eye tracking system, haptic feedback, no port docking, unlimited usage

TABLE 2: Robotic rectal cancer studies in brief.[15]

Author	Study type	Patient numbers	Comparisons	Endpoints
de Jesus et al.	Single-center retrospective	• 59 robotic, 200 open • 41 laparoscopic	Laparoscopic versus robotic versus open total mesorectal excision	Number of LNs, CRM
Cho et al.	Retrospective case-matched study from Yonsei colorectal cancer Database	• 278 laparoscopic • 278 robotic	Robotic versus lap total mesorectal excision	Conversion rates, time to flatus, local recurrence rates, number of LNs, CRM, complications, LOS, five-year survival, DFS
Valverde et al.	Single-center retrospective cohort	• 65 laparoscopic • 65 robotic	Robotic versus laparoscopic sphincter-saving resection for rectal cancer	Morbidity, LOS, conversion rates, quality of TME, CRM, and DRM
Baik et al.[16]	Single-center prospectively randomized	• 57 laparoscopic • 56 robotic	Robotic versus lap low anterior resection	TME quality, operative times, complication rates, conversion rates, CRM involvement

Contd...

Contd...

Author	Study type	Patient numbers	Comparisons	Endpoints
Kim et al.[6]	Single center, prospective cohort	• 39 laparoscopic • 30 robotic	Laparoscopic versus robotic total mesorectal excision	Voiding and sexual function at 1, 6, and 12 months following surgery
Park et al.[17]	Single-center, prospective cohort	• 52 robotic • 88 open • 123 laparoscopic	Laparoscopic versus robotic versus open resection for rectal cancer	Methods of specimen extraction, operating time, LOS, complication rates, number of LNs, CRM, DRM
Somashekhar et al.	Single-center prospective randomized	• 25 open • 25 robotic	Open resection versus robotic for rectal cancer	Operative times, LOS, EBL, conversion rates, DRM, number of LNs, quality TME
D'Annibale et al.[18]	Single-center retrospective	• 50 laparoscopic • 50 robotic	Laparoscopic versus robotic total mesorectal excision	Anastomotic leak rate, operative time, LOS, morbidity, conversion rates, number of LNs, CRM, DRM, urinary and sexual function
Kang et al.	Single-center prospective cohort	• 165 robotic • 165 open • 165 laparoscopic	Laparoscopic versus robotic versus open resection for rectal cancer	LOS, 2-year DFS, voiding, and sexual function, time to flatus, CRM
Feroci et al.	Single-center retrospective	• 58 laparoscopic • 53 robotic	Robotic versus lap total mesorectal excision	LOS, conversion rates, number of LNs, DRM, morbidity, three-year overall survival and DFS

(LOS: length of stay; LN: lymph node; DRM: distal resection margin; DFS: disease-free survival; TME: total mesorectal excision; d: days; EBL: estimated blood loss; LS: laparoscopic surgery; MD: mean difference; RR: risk ratio; CRM: circumferential resection margin; HR: hazard ratio; SMD: standard mean difference; OS: open surgery; OR: odds ratio; SD: standard deviation; RS: robotic surgery)

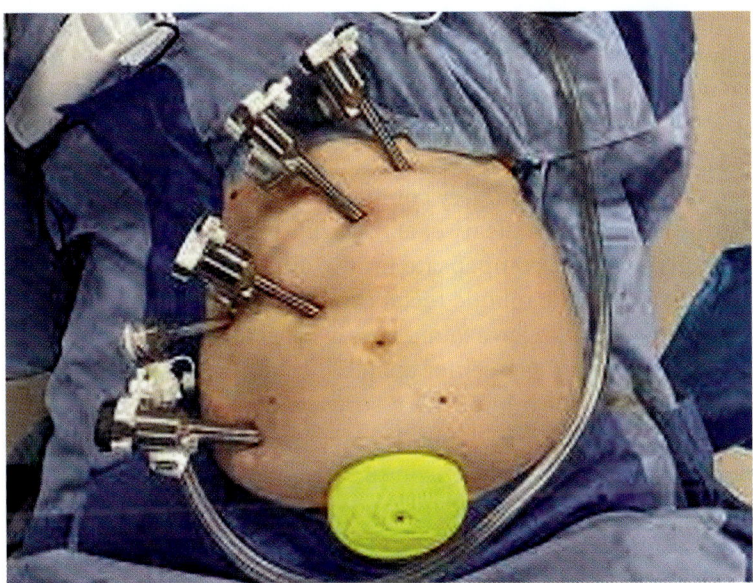

Fig. 1: Port positions for robotic anterior resection with total mesorectal excision (TME).

compared to conventional laparoscopic surgery. This concept has been translated from robotic prostatectomy, where nerve preservation has shown better sexual and urinary function. The largest study of its kind to date, the ROLARR (Robotic vs. Laparoscopic Resection for Rectal Cancer) experiment, was published in 2017.[7] It is a multicenter, randomized controlled trial evaluating the primary endpoint of conversion to laparotomy to carry out TME. Only experienced surgeons in robotics (mean ≥50) and laparoscopy (mean ≥90 prior cases) were included in the study. Surgeons who were in the learning process were eliminated. Evaluation of surgical complications, urinary bladder and sexual dysfunction, mortality, circumferential radial margins (CRMs), and pathologic evaluation of the TME were secondary objectives. No changes in secondary endpoints or conversion rates were observed. It is worth mentioning that robotic surgery extends the length of the operation. The researchers concluded that robots were inappropriate for surgery on rectal cancer, considering the higher expense and nearly identical results.

The ROLARR's results were inconsistent. In an editorial, in contrast to the findings of the CLASICC (conventional versus laparoscopic-assisted surgery in patients with colorectal cancer) trial, Soliman stated that the ROLARR trial was underpowered in terms of conversion rate and surgeon experience and that the study used the third-generation da Vinci Si robot system.[8] According to the data, robotics is more effective in preventing conversion in male patients, obese patients, and those with low tumors. Positive rates of the CRM in the robotic arm (5.1%) were lower compared to the laparoscopic technique, as shown in the CLASICC[9] (7%), ACOSOG Z6051[10] (12%), COLOR II[11] (10%), and AlaCaRT[12] (7%) trials. The outcomes of surgeons lacking robotic case expertise were equal to those of laparoscopic surgeons with two to three times as much expertise. In 2013, Scarpinata and Aly[13] found low conversion to open rates for robotic surgery compared to laparoscopic surgery (1–7.3% vs. 3–22%). According to Cleary et al.,[14] the lower conversion rates in robotic rectal surgeries could compensate for the additional expenses associated with robots. Regarding robotic rectal cancer surgery, several single-center, nonrandomized studies have found positive oncological outcomes.

In Italy, using a single-center analysis, D'Annibale et al. described the oncological results of robotic TME surgery. Out of 100 patients, 50 had laparoscopic TME and 50 had robotic TME. The CRM involvement was none in the robotic group in comparison to <2 mm in six laparoscopic patients ($p = 0.022$). The negative resection margin rate was assumed to be due to the robot's improved ergonomics and visualization. The robotic TME had a higher mean number of extracted lymph nodes (16.5 ± 7.1 vs. 13.8 ± 6.7), although the difference was statistically insignificant ($p = 0.073$). The researchers concluded that robotic TME was more effective and oncologically sound for CRM compared to laparoscopic TME. An earlier study reported that the 3-year overall and 3-year disease-free survival rates were 93.1% and 79.2%, respectively. Local recurrence's 3-year cumulative incidence reached 3.6%, while the CRM positive rate was 5.7%.[16]

In 2010, Pigazzi et al. evaluated 143 patients who had robotic rectal cancer surgery and reported significant short-term clinical results.[19] After a mean follow-up of 17.4 months, there were no local recurrences, and the 3-year survival rate was 97%. This research showed that patients had neoadjuvant chemoradiation; consequently, results should be interpreted carefully. According to this study, robotic surgery would result in higher-quality TME than laparoscopic surgery.

According to D'Annibale et al.,[18] 1-year following resection, only 43% of the sexually active individuals who underwent laparoscopic surgery fully recovered sexual function compared to 100% of patients in the robotic group. Although robotic surgery has been considered safe with a similar complication rate to laparoscopic surgery, Yeo et al.[20] showed increased rates of iatrogenic complications in robotic surgery (OR = 1.73).

Robotic Ventral Mesh Rectopexy (Figs. 2A and B)

Organ prolapse repair in the pelvis via minimal access surgery is challenging. It requires meticulous undistracted dissection, intracorporeal suturing of a mesh to the rectum deep in the pelvis, and vital organ preservation. For such procedures, robotic surgery appears to be an ideal armament. Only three studies[21-23] reporting the ventral mesh robotic rectopexy complication rates

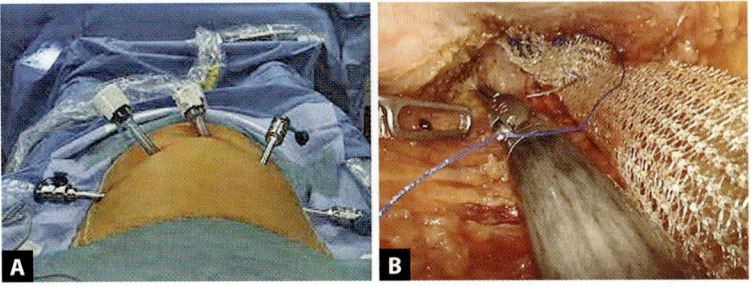

Figs. 2A and B: Port positions of robotic ventral mesh rectopexy (VMR) with mesh being sutured to the sacral promontory.

have been found on comprehensive literature search. These studies have been included in a recent meta-analysis,[24] which revealed that, in comparison to laparoscopic ventral mesh rectopexy (VMR), robotic surgery had an insignificant advantage concerning the intraoperative and postoperative complications including bleeding, vaginal/rectal perforation, autonomic nerve damage, mesh-related complications, postoperative persistence of incontinence, dyspareunia, and constipation. Robotic and laparoscopic VMR procedures were compared in a randomized controlled trial[25] that revealed no significant difference in their complication rates. Concerning functional results following robotic ventral mesh rectopexy (RVMR), significant enhancements in obstructed defecation symptoms were equivalent to those observed following laparoscopic VMR.[23]

Additionally, it has been demonstrated that the two procedures' recurrence rates are comparable. Based on the available data, robotic mesh rectopexy represents a safe surgery with acceptable recurrence rates at 1-year follow-up. However, such a conclusion has some limitations due to the small number of patients included, the short-term follow-up, and the lack of cost-effectiveness data.

Robotic Right Colectomy

The first benign cecal and sigmoid diverticulitis robotic colectomies were documented by Weber et al.[26] Furthermore, Hashizume et al.[27] reported the first malignant disease robotic colectomies. Robotic colectomy has been recognized as the optimal platform for conducting complete mesocolic excision and high central ligation of the colic vessels. Further benefits involve a decreased risk of incisional hernia by avoiding a larger specimen extraction site and easier intracorporeal anastomosis. In a case–control study of cancer patients, Morpurgo et al.[28] compared laparoscopic extracorporeal anastomosis ($n = 48$) with robotic intracorporeal anastomosis ($n = 48$). The researchers demonstrated shorter hospital stay (7.5 ± 2.0 vs. 9.0 ± 3.2 days, respectively; $p < 0.05$), rapid recovery of bowel function (3 ± 1 vs. 4.0 days, respectively; $p < 0.05$), fewer anastomotic leaks, and fewer incisional hernias (0 vs. 4 and 0 vs. 4, respectively). Their conclusion was that patients who underwent intracorporeal robotic anastomosis had faster recovery than those subjected to extracorporeal laparoscopic anastomosis. In a recent meta-analysis, Xu et al.[29] compared both laparoscopic and robotic right hemicolectomy. The study included one randomized controlled trial and six nonrandomized trials. Out of 649 participants enrolled in these trials, 234 were subjected to robotic surgeries and 415 were operated on with laparoscopic techniques. According to the findings, robotic right colectomies required a longer time, but they were associated with faster bowel function recovery, shorter hospital stay, lesser estimated blood losses, and fewer overall postoperative complications. However, robotic right hemicolectomy has several limitations including its higher cost, longer operating duration, and lack of considerable patients' benefits over laparoscopic surgery.

■ COST ANALYSIS OF ROBOTIC SURGERY

The robot's cost represents a frequently discussed topic. However, when attempting to put a value on its utility, it is essential to comprehend the mechanisms of the robotic price tag. According to the 2017 Intuitive Surgical Annual Report and data acquired from the American Hospital Association, around 4,400 da Vinci systems were found worldwide in 2017, with approximately 2,800 of the 5,500 (51%) United States hospitals having a robotic presence (up from 27% in 2012). In the same year, approximately 644,000 robotic surgeries were carried out in the United States, with general surgery incorporating colorectal surgery having the fastest-growing market (and the third-largest overall market, after urology and gynecology). In 2017, a da Vinci robot's average sales price was $1.47 million, with yearly servicing contracts costing between $80,000 and $170,000.[30] According to Feldstein et al.,[30] maintenance costs, variable case costs for services or procedures (time, materials, staff), and the cost of initial equipment acquisition could all be added together to determine how much it would cost to own a da Vinci robot. The authors provided information indicating that the typical robot in the USA executes 424 cases per year and that the robot has an average fixed cost of $948 per use. Each procedure's weighted cost ranged from $3,325, for a cholecystectomy, to $16,986, for a rectal excision, with an average of $8,025. According to estimations within 14 facilities for high-volume robotics (rural, academic, and community), a single rectal resection costs $17,970 overall. Even after insurance payments, data from earlier randomized controlled trials indicated that robotic colonic resection was significantly more expensive than laparoscopic resection.[17,31]

■ ONGOING RESEARCH

Robotic telementoring is the use of the robotic platform to allow the remote presence of an expert during a trainee's performance of a complicated clinical task, such as an operation or management of a critically ill patient. The term "telementoring" suggests a structured teaching role, which distinguishes it from robotic teleconsultation which is the use of a robotic platform to provide on-demand expert opinion for specific complex clinical scenarios in a remote area. Schlachta and colleagues have demonstrated that a structured mentoring and telementoring model can be used to transfer and incorporate laparoscopic colon surgery from a university center to a community setting.[32] The telementoring in their model was conducted via an internet protocol point-to-point connection, by which the mentor witnessed the robotic colon surgery. The mentor could provide verbal guidance as well as be able to draw on a touchscreen with a stylus to create an overlay diagram that the operating surgeon (trainee) could see on his screen which would help him in the performance of safe and efficient surgery.

Image Integration in Robotics

Navigation for current robotic-assisted surgical techniques is primarily accomplished through a stereo pair of endoscopic camera images. These images provide standard optical visualization of the surface but provide no subsurface information. Image guidance methods allow the visualization of subsurface information such as the position of tumor margins or vascular structures which is crucial in delivering appropriate and safe treatment. Herrell et al. in 2008 at the Vanderbilt University (Tennessee, USA) validated a system which integrated CT imaging with a da Vinci® S system and used it on gel blocks which were simulated to mimic tumors.[33] The preoperative CT images were continually streamed into the surgeon console. The view could be toggled between a pure camera image and the split screen by a tap on the camera pedal. This configuration allowed the surgeon to augment the current technique with the additional information provided by the image integration system. However spatial, technological and financial constraints limit the development of such versatile robotic systems. MRI and CT-guided systems remain as an item of interest under constant advancement; currently, these systems are still experimental.

■ PATIENT-SPECIFIC SURGERY IN ROBOTICS

Although underlying colorectal pathology such as tumors may be the same across patients, the presentation and interventional approach to treat varies from patient to patient. Hence, it is logical to develop patient-specific surgical robotic systems with arms specifically designed and constructed for colorectal manipulation or retraction or bowel stapling to maximize the benefits of robot-assisted surgery. But manufacturing patient-specific robots can be challenging for complex procedures such as pelvic exenteration. They are also expensive, time consuming to construct, and cannot be used on other patients as they are specifically designed for a certain patient for a specific treatment. 3D printing can help to mitigate this issue.

■ CONCLUSION

As eager, younger surgeons enter today's surgical workforce, they train with the aim to be technically proficient and efficient in minimally invasive approaches. Current evidence indicates that robotic surgery is noninferior to laparoscopic surgery in colorectal cancer and rectal prolapse with cost being the only issue. As technology and the market share for robotics continue to diversify and grow, the costs should hopefully improve. With evolution, surgeons will be able to offer "patient-specific" surgery to reduce complications with improved short- and long-term outcomes.

■ REFERENCES

1. Giulianotti PC, Coratti A, Angelini M, Sbrana F, Cecconi S, Balestracci T, et al. Robotics in general surgery: personal experience in a large community hospital. Arch Surg. 2003;138(7):777-84.
2. Ngu JC, Tsang CB, Koh DC. The da Vinci Xi: a review of its capabilities, versatility, and potential role in robotic colorectal surgery. Robot Surg. 2017;4:77-85.
3. Hance J, Rockall T, Darzi A. Robotics in colorectal surgery. Dig Surg. 2004;21: 339-43.
4. Lanfranco AR, Castellanos AE, Desai JP, Meyers WC. Robotic surgery: a current perspective. Ann Surg. 2004;239:14-21.
5. Pigazzi A, Ellenhorn JD, Ballantyne GH, Paz IB. Robotic-assisted laparoscopic low anterior resection with total mesorectal excision for rectal cancer. Surg Endosc. 2006;20:1521-5.
6. Kim CW, Kim CH, Baik SH. Outcomes of robotic-assisted colorectal surgery compared with laparoscopic and open surgery: a systematic review. J Gastrointest Surg. 2014;18:816-30.
7. Jayne D, Pigazzi A, Marshall H, Croft J, Corrigan N, Copeland J, et al. Effect of robotic-assisted vs. conventional laparoscopic surgery on risk of conversion to open laparotomy among patients undergoing resection for rectal cancer: The ROLARR randomized clinical trial. JAMA. 2017;318:1569-80.
8. Soliman M. (2017). ROLARR—the real story. [online] Available from: https://www.linkedin.com/pulse/rolarr-real-story-mark-soliman-md-facs-fascrs [Last accessed November, 2022].
9. Guillou PJ, Quirke P, Thorpe H, Walker J, Jayne DG, Smith AMH, et al. Short-term endpoints of conventional versus laparoscopic-assisted surgery in patients with colorectal cancer (MRC CLASICC trial): multicentre, randomised controlled trial. Lancet. 2005;365:1718-26.
10. Fleshman J, Branda ME, Sargent DJ, Boller AM, George VV, Abbas MA, et al. Disease-free survival and local recurrence for laparoscopic resection compared with open resection of stage II to III rectal cancer: Follow-up results of the ACOSOG Z6051 randomized controlled trial. Ann Surg. 2019;269:589-95.
11. van der Pas MH, Haglind E, Cuesta MA, Fürst A, Lacy AM, Hop WC, et al. Laparoscopic versus open surgery for rectal cancer (COLOR II): short-term outcomes of a randomised, phase 3 trial. Lancet Oncol. 2013;14:210-8.

12. Stevenson AR, Solomon MJ, Lumley JW, Hewett P, Clouston AD, Gebski VJ, et al. Effect of laparoscopic-assisted resection vs. open resection on pathological outcomes in rectal cancer: The ALaCaRT Randomized Clinical Trial. JAMA. 2015;314:1356-63.
13. Scarpinata R, Aly EH. Does robotic rectal cancer surgery offer improved early postoperative outcomes? Dis Colon Rectum. 2013;56(2):253-62.
14. Cleary RK, Mullard AJ, Ferraro J, Regenbogen SE. The cost of conversion in robotic and laparoscopic colorectal surgery. Surg Endosc. 2018;32(3):1515-24.
15. Cheng CL, Rezac C. The role of robotics in colorectal surgery. BMJ. 2018;360:j5304.
16. Baik SH, Kim NK, Lim DR, Min BS, Lee KY. Oncologic outcomes and perioperative clinicopathologic results after robot-assisted tumor-specific mesorectal excision for rectal cancer. Ann Surg Oncol. 2013;20(8):2625-32.
17. Park JS, Choi GS, Park SY, Kim HJ, Ryuk JP. Randomized clinical trial of robot-assisted versus standard laparoscopic right colectomy. Br J Surg. 2012;99:1219-26.
18. D'Annibale A, Pernazza G, Monsellato I, Pinde V, Lucandri G, Mazzocchi P, et al. Total mesorectal excision: a comparison of oncological and functional outcomes between robotic and laparoscopic surgery for rectal cancer. Surg Endosc. 2013;27(6):1887-95.
19. Pigazzi A, Luca F, Patriti A, Valvo M, Ceccarelli G, Casciola L, et al. Multicentric study on robotic tumor-specific mesorectal excision for the treatment of rectal cancer. Ann Surg Oncol. 2010;17(6):1614-20.
20. Yeo HL, Isaacs AJ, Abelson JS, Milsom JW, Sedrakyan A. Comparison of open, laparoscopic, and robotic colectomies using a large national database: outcomes and trends related to surgery center volume. Dis Colon Rectum. 2016;59(6):535-42.
21. Mäkelä-Kaikkonen J, Rautio T, Klintrup K, Takala H, Vierimaa M, et al. Robotic assisted and laparoscopic ventral rectopexy in the treatment of rectal prolapse: a matched-pairs study of operative details and complications. Tech Coloproctol. 2014;18(2):151-5.
22. Wong MT, Meurette G, Rigaud J, Regenet N. Robotic versus laparoscopic rectopexy for complex rectocele: a prospective comparison of short term outcomes. Dis Colon Rectum. 2011;54(3):342-6.
23. Mantoo S, Podevin J, Regenet N, Rigaud J, Lehur PA, Meurette G. Is robotic-assisted ventral mesh rectopexy superior to laparoscopic ventral mesh rectopexy in the management of obstructed defaecation. Colorectal Dis. 2013;15(8):e469-75.
24. van Iersel JJ, Paulides TJ, Verheijen PM, Lumley JW, Broeders IAMJ, Consten ECJ. Current status of laparoscopic and robotic ventral mesh rectopexy for external and internal rectal prolapse. World J Gastroenterol. 2016;22(21):4977-87.
25. Mäkelä-Kaikkonen J, Rautio T, Pääkkö E, Biancari F, Ohtonen P, Mäkelä J. Robot assisted vs. laparoscopic ventral rectopexy for external or internal rectal prolapse and enterocele: a randomised controlled trial. Colorectal Dis. 2016;18(10):1010-5.
26. Weber PA, Merola S, Wasielewski A, Ballantyne GH. Telerobotic-assisted laparoscopic right and sigmoid colectomies for benign disease. Dis Colon Rectum. 2002;45(12):1689-94; discussion 95-96.
27. Hashizume M, Shimada M, Tomikawa M, Ikeda Y, Takahashi I, Abe R, et al. Early experiences of endoscopic procedures in general surgery assisted by a computer-enhanced surgical system. Surg Endosc. 2002;16(8):1187-91.

28. Morpurgo E, Contardo T, Molaro R, Zerbinati A, Orisini C, D'Annibale A. Robotic-assisted intracorporeal anastomosis versus extracorporeal anastomosis in laparoscopic right hemicolectomy for cancer: a case control study. J Laparoendosc Advs Surg Tech A. 2013;23(5):414-7.
29. Xu H, Li J, Sun Y, Li Z, Zhen Y, Wag B, Xu Z. Robotic versus laparoscopic right colectomy: a metaanalysis. World J Surg Oncol. 2014;12:274.
30. Feldstein J, Schwander B, Roberts M, Coussons H. Cost of ownership assessment for a da Vinci robot based on US real-world data. Int J Med Robot. 2019;15: e2023.
31. Ma S, Chen Y, Chen Y, Guo T, Yang X, Lu Y, et al. Short-term outcomes of robotic-assisted right colectomy compared with laparoscopic surgery: A systematic review and meta-analysis. Asian J Surg. 2019;42:589-98.
32. Schlachta CM, Sorsdahl AK, Lefebvre KL, McCune ML, Jayaraman S.A model for longitudinal mentoring and telementoring of laparoscopic colon surgery. Surg Endosc. 2009;23(7):1634-8.
33. Herrell SD, Kwartowitz D, Milhoua PM, Galloway RL. Toward image guided robotic surgery: system validation. J Urol. 2008;181(2):783-9.

8 Robotic Transoral Surgery

Kalpana Nagpal

■ INTRODUCTION

Interest in functional organ preservation surgery (FOPS) has risen significantly over the past few years, as clinicians and researchers attempt to increase overall survival, functional outcomes, and quality of life (QoL), while reducing the adverse effects of treatment.

Transoral robotic surgery (TORS), as an organ preserving modality, is becoming more popular, and the potential of expanding indications for future applications, with the introduction of new robots and integrated imaging, will play a crucial role in its adoption. Transoral robotic surgery can play an important role in the management of carcinoma of unknown primary (CUP) as tongue base mucosectomy has been included in the National Institute for Health and Care Excellence (NICE) guidelines for the evaluation of CUP, if FDG PET-CT (fluorodeoxyglucose positron emission tomography-computed tomography) does not identify a possible primary site.

Transoral robotic surgery is a modern, minimally invasive procedure, using robotic technology that enables surgery of lesions in the oral cavity, pharynx, larynx, base of the skull and neck, via direct access through a natural orifice, the mouth, i.e., Robotic Natural Orifice Transluminal Endoscopic Surgery (R-NOTES).

Transoral robotic sleep apnea (TORSA) surgery uses the same approach to treat patients of obstructive sleep apnea (OSA), in patients who do not tolerate continuous positive airway pressure (CPAP), and also in patients who do not benefit from conventional (nonrobotic) surgery for OSA.

Transoral robotic thyroidectomy (TORT) is a novel technique for minimally invasive thyroid surgery.

Transoral robotic reconstruction surgery (TORRS) has emerged as a technique for reconstruction of defects after surgery with free flaps and transfer of adjacent tissue.

The classification system for transoral oropharyngeal defects maps defects into four classes and guides the reconstructive thought process.

The available reconstructive options allow an expanding role of this minimally invasive surgery, even in locally advanced tumors.

■ HISTORICAL OVERVIEW

The origin of TORS can be traced to the publication of a case report in 2005, of robotic transoral supraglottic partial laryngectomy in a canine model, using the da Vinci Surgical Robot, and the first clinical report by McLeod and Melder of a da Vinci-assisted excision of a vallecular cyst, after a review of the potential applications of the Da Vinci minimally invasive surgical robotic system in otolaryngology, in porcine and cadaveric models.

The pioneering team of Professors Gregory Weinstein and Bert O'Malley, Jr, at the University of Pennsylvania, was instrumental in getting Food and Drug Administration (FDA) approval of TORS, for the management of early stage (T1 and T2) head and neck cancer in 2009.

Transoral robotic surgery as a multilevel treatment modality for the management of obstructive sleep apnea–hypopnea syndrome (OSAHS) was first described by Professor Claudio Vicini et al. in 2010 at Forli, Italy.

■ ROBOTIC PLATFORM

The da Vinci Robotic Surgical System, with multijointed instruments having EndoWrist technology, and innovative cameras with advanced digital optics, enables precise magnified three-dimensional high-definition (3DHD) visualization for robotic-assisted TORS, with true depth perception and precision surgery, in difficult to access areas and tight surgical spaces.

The da Vinci Surgical System consists of a surgeon console from which commands are relayed via cables to the patient side cart located near the patient. The surgeon sits at a computer console controlling a robotic camera, and performs robotic-assisted surgery using robotic arms that match the surgeon's hand movements precisely, with the help of an assistant surgeon, at the operation table next to the patient, for suction, traction, and management of the patient.

The surgeon controls the movement of the endoscopic instruments and the camera with two master tool manipulators. The endoscopic instruments and the endoscope are held in a fixed position with respect to the patient, by two or three patient side manipulators, and the endoscope camera manipulator, respectively. Commands from the surgeon console are relayed to the patient side cart via cables. Instrument and endoscope changes are performed by an assistant who is positioned near the patient side cart. The Insite Vision System combines two independent images to form a 2D or 3D image of the surgical field, which is relayed to the surgeon seated at the surgeon console. The FDA approved the use of the da Vinci Surgical System for Transoral Otolaryngology procedures in 2009 and it is currently the global market leader for TORS.

The first application of the Medrobotics Flex^{TM} System in human beings was an assessment of the safety profile, functionality, and ease of use for

TORS at a tertiary referral unit by Professor Marc Remacle et al. in 2015. It consists of a flexible endoscope with articulated segments, specifically designed for TORS, and has been approved for use in the European and US markets since 2016.

Innovative single port (SP) technology has transformed TORS in 2019. The da Vinci SP system has a single 2.5 cm port through which three fully-wristed, elbowed 6 mm instruments and the first fully-wristed da Vinci 1.2 cm stereo endoscope camera are used.

Indications

Indications include:
- Benign and malignant tumors of oropharynx, including advanced oropharyngeal carcinoma (benefit of lower gastrostomy dependency rates)
- Benign tumors and lesions of the parapharyngeal space, accessible from the oropharynx, with no carotid encasement or bone erosion
- **Transoral robotic** surgery supraglottic laryngectomy (TORS-SL) (no patients required tracheostomy or gastrostomy)
- **Transoral robotic total laryngectomy (TL) or TORS-assisted TL in selected cases like recurrence or post-therapeutic organ dysfunction (no patient needed gastrostomy supplementation)**
- *Hypopharyngeal lesions:* Transoral robotic medial hypopharyngectomy was described in 2016, and single-port transoral robotic surgery (SP TORS) hypopharyngectomy was considered for resectable hypopharyngeal tumors in 2021, since they can be reached and successfully treated with the improved flexibility and access of the SP robotic system by adjustments of the semiflexible endoscope and use of the third transoral surgical instrumentation.
- TORS BOT (base of tongue) mucosectomy is a safe and useful procedure in the diagnostic and therapeutic workup for CUP in an era of increasing incidence of human papillomavirus (HPV)-positive OPSCC (oropharyngeal squamous cell carcinoma).
- TORSA surgery for OSAHS (in patients not tolerating CPAP) with appropriate patient selection.
- Pediatric TORS procedures are safe and feasible and have been demonstrated up to the laryngeal region.
- Robot-assisted reconstruction of defects with free flaps.
- Transoral robotic nasopharyngectomy for recurrent nasopharyngeal cancer after radiotherapy (RT).
- TORS for sellar tumors.
- TORS-assisted sialolithotomy.

"Pearls" of Transoral Robotic Surgery and How I Do It

- Operating the surgeon console is the same with both Si and Xi systems.
- Anesthesia machine should be near the foot end in TORS cases.
- Nasal intubation (flexometallic tube) is most preferable in TORS cases.
- Having a good retractor which can give maximum mouth opening as well that can retract cheeks is required.
- If you are not ready with everything, do not use the retractor and keep the mouth open for too long, as this can cause bluish discoloration of the tongue and edema.
- Before you remove the instruments from the instrument arms or undock they have to be straightened, otherwise the tips may break **(Fig. 1)**.
- The amount of extension required of the neck depends on the area you want to operate: for tongue base extension required will be different from larynx cases.
- Additional horizontal cuts shall be parallel to the initial cut at the foremen cecum.
- The dissection goes in a step ladder fashion till a trough is created.
- All this is for sleep apnea.
- For cancers wide resection is planned.
- Patient side assistant should be well trained to provide the primary surgeon with a good field.
- Avoid TORS in patients with trismus and in patients where cervical extension is not possible.

This is just the beginning of advanced technologies that will keep increasing in the coming years. Surgical methods will keep evolving

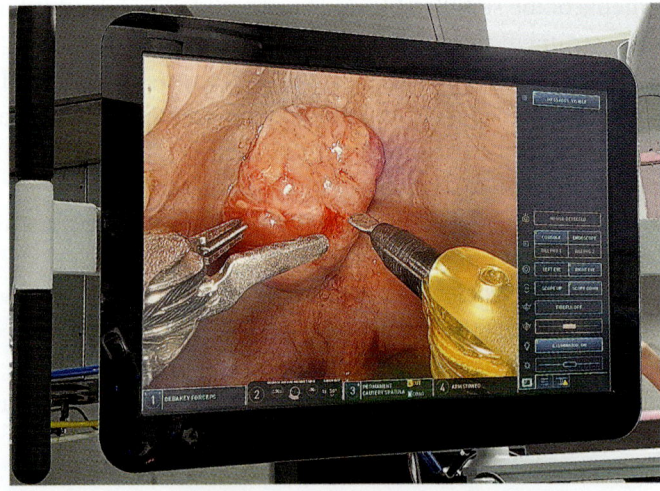

Fig. 1: Transoral robotic surgery.

and robotic technology too. Our society is slowly accepting the change. Based upon the outcomes patients have now a good option. There is lack of awareness and even if there is one, there is more negativity than positivity probably because traditional surgeons are significantly more in numbers. The working angles provided with robotic technology is amazing and one needs to actually experience this to appreciate it.

Informed Consent

The presence of "Preceptor" and "Proctor" should be indicated, and responsibilities must be made clear for the informed consent, with incorporation of data about the surgeon's experience in TORS, and the number of procedures of the department. Informed consent is shifting toward a more appropriate concept of defensive-informed consent.

Docking

Positioning of the operation table, including the tilt of the table, is done in accordance with surgeon preference, depending on the procedure, before docking the robotic arms. The operation table should not be moved after the robotic patient side cart is positioned and the instrument arms are placed in their appropriate positions inside the oral cavity **(Fig. 2)**.

There is no single method for determining the optimal position of ports, as the port position may differ depending on the surgeon, the procedure, and the patient. It is difficult to develop guidelines for

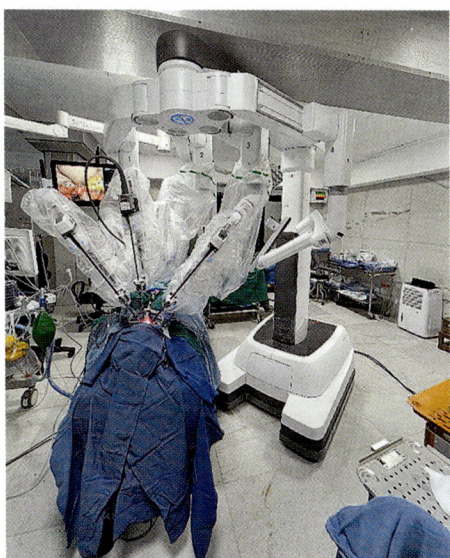

Fig. 2: Docking of the da Vinci surgical system for transoral robotic surgery (TORS) with the camera arm and two robotic instrument arms.

specific port placement, but broad guidelines are based on maximizing the view from the endoscope and the reach of the instruments, while simultaneously minimizing the clashes between the arms.

The 12 mm camera arm is inserted in the midline through the mouth gag, with the cannula tip in the oral cavity, and the camera is adjusted so that it is parallel to the tongue blade, and advanced to the desired position. The 5 mm instrument arms are positioned with the thick black line outside, and the tip of the cannula at the level of the mouth gag, with the angle adjusted so that the instruments are visualized just beyond the tip of the endoscope. The cutting tool in the instrument arm can be the original unipolar electrocautery in TORS-EC or the laser in TORS-L (flexible carbon dioxide laser in CO_2-TORS, or diode thulium: yttrium aluminum garnet (YAG) laser in TY-TORS) and is conventionally placed on the side of the lesion, with the tissue holding forceps placed on the contralateral side.

Good "docking" makes the surgery easier to perform and gives better outcomes.

Advantage over Open Surgery

Transoral robotic surgery is a treatment modality which offers a number of advantages over open surgery and has emerged as an alternative to open surgery and/or nonsurgical treatment with its multiple benefits **(Box 1)**.

Benefit of Transoral Robotic Surgery

The benefit of TORS for the patient includes reduced blood loss during surgery, with better cosmetic results and function preservation, minimized morbidity with decreased postoperative pain and chance of wound infection, leading to improved QoL and outcomes like short hospital stay,

BOX 1: Advantage of transoral robotic surgery (TORS) over open surgery.

- Minimally invasive approach
- Natural orifice access avoids incision and scar
- Reduced surgeon fatigue due to console ergonomics
- Avoid mandibulotomy/pharyngotomy and tracheostomy
- Precision surgery
- Panoramic view
- Image magnification
- 3D visualization
- Motion scaling
- Tremor reduction
- 7 degrees of freedom of instruments
- Overcomes line of sight restriction
- Telesurgery

quick recovery, and early return to normal activity, including speech and swallowing, with minimal scarring.

Patients with head and neck cancer may have the added advantage of avoiding the side effects of chemotherapy and/or RT, and in selected cases de-escalation of cancer treatment may be possible with good functional and oncological outcomes.

ANESTHESIA PERIOPERATIVE MANAGEMENT

For transoral robotic surgery the anesthetist should be able to handle difficult intubations. Good experienced anesthetist is required to do nasal intubation. A north facing tube is required. Pre- and post-operative pain management and other anesthetic challenges are well known. These cases are therefore to be done in big hospitals with a good back up.

Complications of TORS
- Mucosal injury to lips and cheeks
- Dental injury
- Bleeding ranging from minor to torrential
- Loss of taste
- Dysphagia ranging for a few days to weeks
- Need for a tracheostomy due to postoperative edema
- Pharyngocutaneous fistula
- Pharyngeal stricture and velopharyngeal insufficiency
- TMJ dislocation rarely because of forcefully opening the mouth using retractors .

TORS during COVID-19 Pandemic

Guidelines recommend triage of otolaryngology patients with provision of, time sensitive and emergency, office-based and surgical care, in order to reduce the risk of transmission of the severe acute respiratory syndrome coronavirus 2 (SARS-CoV-2) from human to human during the coronavirus disease 2019 (COVID-19) pandemic. Renin–angiotensin system (RAS) in ear, nose, and throat (ENT) and head and neck surgery can effectively minimize the risk of contamination of healthcare providers, as compared to open approaches. Use of adequate personal protective equipment (PPE) and preventing the release of surgical smoke leak offer a safe surgical environment for both the patient and the surgical team.

Transoral robotic surgery has the advantage of maintaining distance between the surgeon, the patient, and other staff of the hospital during the current COVID-19 pandemic scenario, resulting in a lower risk of transmission of the virus as compared to open surgery. It obviates the need for procedures like tracheostomy and mandibulotomy which are associated with aerosol generation. TORS minimizes the risk of direct exposure of healthcare providers to smoke, gases, body fluids, and aerosols generated by surgery. It is essential to have a safe and effective method to vent smoke and gas generated during surgery.

The use of sterile plastic drapes with water-tight seal around each robotic cannula can help reduce viral transmission to healthcare providers during TORS.

A transparent plastic bag can be unrolled to cover and wrap the nose and mouth of the patient (including retractor) during TORS with small holes made for the endoscope, robotic instrument arms, and suction.

The Negative-pressure Otolaryngology Viral Isolation Drape (NOVID) system was introduced to minimize aerosol and droplet contamination. It consists of a plastic drape suspended above the patient's head with a smoke evacuator suction placed inside the chamber.

Povidone-iodine-I (PVP-I) solutions are virucidal against related coronaviruses, relatively safe to use in the upper airway, require very brief application times, and may potentially reduce the risk of SARS-CoV-2 aerosolization and transmission during upper airway mucosal surgery.

WHO, Centers for Disease Control and Prevention (CDC), and Centre for Health Protection (CHP) recommend full barrier protection to avoid disease transmission to healthcare providers. Such PPE includes gloves, goggles, face shield, and gowns, as well as items filtering facepiece respirators such as N95 or powered air-purifying respirator (PAPR) hoods and aprons.

To reduce the risk of viral transmission and conserve PPE at times of global shortage, the number of healthcare providers within the operating theater is kept at a minimum at all times.

In view of COVID-19 pandemic, there have been many guidelines and protocols on how to manage the airway, intubate, and perform tracheostomy for unknown, suspected, and confirmed COVID-19 patients.

To minimize aerosol exposure, complete paralysis of the patient must be ascertained throughout the procedure; mechanical ventilation is stopped prior to tracheotomy; tracheotomy is performed using scalpel knife; suction is not to be used during and after tracheotomy; all tracheostomies are to be performed by one consultant surgeon, one consultant anesthetist, and one scrub nurse experienced in the management of airways and the procedure. Thorough communication before and during the procedure is essential to ensure swift and bloodless execution whilst minimizing aerosol generation.

Other than full barrier protection for all parties, we make use of a clear sterile plastic drape suspended over two horizontal anesthetic screens to create a spacious sterile working "box" in which the surgeon performs tracheostomy. The "plastic box" acts as an additional physical barrier, further protecting the surgeon and healthcare providers in the operating theater against droplet and aerosol contamination. Such a setup is functional, readily available, and cost effective. With such a setup, face shield can be spared for the surgeon and scrub nurse.

■ RESEARCH

Transoral robotic surgery seems to be useful and safe for the diagnosis and management of CUP in the head and neck, in the current scenario of increasing incidence of HPV-positive OPSCC.

De-escalation of adjuvant treatment for HPV+ oropharyngeal cancer: TORS and Eastern Cooperative Oncology Group (ECOG) 3311. Primary transoral surgery and reduced-dose postoperative RT retained outstanding oncologic outcome at 35 months follow-up, with favorable QoL and functional outcomes, in intermediate risk HPV+ oropharynx cancer.

Ongoing Randomized Controlled Trials

Multicenter randomized controlled trials (RCTs) are currently in the recruitment stage. These include the PATHOS (Postoperative Adjuvant Treatment for Human Papillomavirus (HPV)-positive Tumors) trial for HPV-positive oropharyngeal cancer (UK), the RTOG (Radiation Therapy Oncology Group) 1221 trial for HPV-negative oropharyngeal cancer (USA), and the ORATOR study for early-stage oropharyngeal cancer (Canada).

■ TRAINING AND CREDENTIALING

Robotic surgery, across all specialties, continues to be hampered by the absence of a well-defined learning curve (LC), and consensus on the requisite certification necessary to be considered a robotic surgeon.

An international consensus statement on structured robotic surgical training, with defined curricula in different surgical subspecialties, including both technical and nontechnical skills, and implementation according to the IDEAL (Idea, Development, Exploration, Assessment, and Long-term monitoring) framework is the need of the hour for regulated uptake of robot-assisted surgery. Telementoring and simulation training with systems thinking and credentialing with a proficiency-based progression approach will provide an affordable solution. The training curriculum for trainees should proceed along a stepwise, competency-based platform which starts with didactic learning and simulation exercises, and progresses to operative experience, and should include formal evaluation of nontechnical skills like troubleshooting of robotic surgical systems.

Dr Kalpana Nagpal mentors surgeons for certification in head and neck robotic surgery in India.

■ MARKET AND COST CHALLENGES

Robotic surgery is evolving and indications are expanding and the robots that are being made currently have additional features but in India cost factor remains a hurdle. The volumes could have been much more. Robotic surgeons in the field of ENT and Head Neck surgery are very few and make in India robot has just been launched. Other robots are very expensive including the cost of consumables. There is a huge potential and huge market for people who want to invest.

■ FUTURE APPLICATIONS

Current developments of new, flexible surgical robots will not only improve outcomes and safety for patients, but will also result in cheaper and cost-effective treatment for an increasing number of indications like lesions in the nasopharynx and glottic area of the larynx, etc.

Future directions relate to overlay technology through augmented reality (AR) that allows real-time image-guidance, miniaturization (nanorobots), and the development of autonomous robots.

■ SUGGESTED READING

1. Centre for Health Protection. (2022). Key Elements on Prevention and Control of Coronavirus Disease (COVID-19) in Healthcare Settings (Interim). [online] Available from: https://www.chp.gov.hk/files/pdf/ic_advice_for_nid_in_healthcare_setting.pdf [Last accessed December, 2022].
2. Chauvet D, Missistrano A, Hivelin M, Carpentier A, Cornu P, Hans S. Transoral robotic-assisted skull base surgery to approach the sella turcica: cadaveric study. Neurosurg Rev. 2014;37(4):609-17.
3. Chauvet D Hans S. Transoral robotic surgery applied to the skull base. In: Assaad F, Wassmann H, Khodor MM (Eds). Pituitary Diseases. London: IntechOpen; 2019.
4. Choo JM, You JY, Kim HY. Transoral robotic thyroidectomy: The overview and suggestions for future research in new minimally invasive thyroid surgery. J Minim Invasive Surg. 2019;22(1):5-10.
5. Chow VL, Chan JY, Wong MM, Wong ST, Tsang RK Novel approach to reduce SAR-CoV-2 transmission during trans-oral robotic surgery. J Robot Surg. 2021;15(6):963-70.
6. Chow VLY. Tracheostomy during COVID-19 pandemic–a novel approach. Authorea. 2020.
7. David AP, Jiam NT, Reither JM, Gurrola JG 2nd, Aghi MK, El-Sayed IH. Endoscopic skull base and transoral surgery during COVID-19 pandemic: Minimizing droplet spread with negative-pressure otolaryngology viral isolation drape. Head Neck. 2020;42(7):1577-82.
8. de Almeida JR, Park RC, Villanueva NL, Miles BA, Teng MS, Genden EM. Reconstructive algorithm and classification system for transoral oropharyngeal defects. Head Neck. 2014;36(7):934-41.

9. Ferrarese A, Pozzi G, Borghi F, Pellegrino L, Di Lorenzo P, Amato B, et al. Informed consent in robotic surgery: quality of information and patient perception. Open Med (Wars). 2016;11(1):279-85.
10. Ferris RL, Flamand Y, Weinstein GS, Shuli Li S, Quon H, Mehra R, et al. Updated report of a phase II randomized trial of transoral surgical resection followed by low-dose or standard postoperative therapy in resectable p16+ locally advanced oropharynx cancer: a trial of the ECOG-ACRIN cancer research group (E3311). J Clin Oncol. 2021;39(15 suppl):6010-10.
11. Garas G, Arora A: Robotic Head and Neck Surgery: History, Technical Evolution and the Future. ORL J Otorhinolaryngol Relat Spec. 2018;80(3-4):117-24.
12. Heyd CP, Desiato VM, Nguyen SA, O'Rourke AK, Clemmens CS, Awad MI, et al. Tracheostomy protocols during COVID-19 pandemic. Head Neck. 2020;42(6):1297-302.
13. McLeod IK, Mair EA, Melder PC. Potential applications of the da Vinci minimally invasive surgical robotic system in otolaryngology. Ear Nose Throat J. 2005;84(8):483-7.
14. McLeod IK, Melder PC. Da Vinci robot-assisted excision of a vallecular cyst: a case report. Ear Nose Throat J. 2005;84(3):170-2.
15. Meccariello G, Cammaroto G, Iannella G, Capaccio P, Pelucchi S, Vicini C. Minimizing contagion risks of COVID-19 during transoral robotic surgery. Laryngoscope. 2020;130(11):2593-4.
16. Meccariello G, Montevecchi F, Sgarzani R, Vicini C. Defect-oriented reconstruction after transoral robotic surgery for oropharyngeal cancer: a case series and review of the literature. Acta Otorhinolaryngol Ital. 2018;38(6): 569-74.
17. Mendelsohn AH, Lawson G. Single-port transoral robotic surgery hypopharyngectomy. Head Neck. 2021;43(10):3234-7.
18. Mendelsohn AH, Remacle M, Van Der Vorst S, Bachy V, Lawson G. Outcomes following transoral robotic surgery: supraglottic laryngectomy. Laryngoscope. 2013;123(1):208-14.
19. Nagpal K, Malik NU, Naruka SS, Rana N. Robotic surgery in ENT and head and neck during the COVID-19 pandemic. Apollo Med. 2020;17(Suppl S1):18-20.
20. National Institute for Health and Care Excellence. (2016). Cancer of the upper aerodigestive tract: assessment and management in people aged 16 and over. [online] Available from: https://www.nice.org.uk/guidance/ng36/chapter/Recommendations [Last accessed December, 2022].
21. O'Malley BW Jr, Quon H, Leonhardt FD, Chalian AA, Weinstein GS. Transoral robotic surgery for parapharyngeal space tumors. ORL J Otorhinolaryngol Relat Spec. 2010;72(6):332-6.
22. Parhar HS, Tasche K, Brody RM, Weinstein GS, O'Malley BW Jr, Shanti RM, et al. Topical preparations to reduce SARS-CoV-2 aerosolization in head and neck mucosal surgery. Head Neck. 2020;42(6):1268-72.
23. Remacle M, MN Prasad V, Lawson G, Plisson L, Bachy V, Van der Vorst S. Transoral robotic surgery (TORS) with the Medrobotics Flex System: first surgical application on humans. Eur Arch Otorhinolaryngol. 2015;272(6):1451-5.
24. Selber JC, Sarhane KA, Ibrahim AE, Holsinger FC. Transoral robotic reconstructive surgery. Semin Plast Surg. 2014;28(1):35-8.

25. Selber JC. Transoral robotic reconstruction of oropharyngeal defects: a case series. Plast Reconstr Surg. 2010;126(6):1978-87.
26. Sharma A, Bhardwaj R. Robotic Surgery in Otolaryngology During the Covid-19 Pandemic: A Safer Approach? Indian J Otolaryngol Head Neck Surg. 2021.;73(1):120-3.
27. Siegel JD, Rhinehart E, Jackson M, Chiarello L; the Healthcare Infection Control Practices Advisory Committee. (2007). Guideline for Isolation Precautions. Part III: Precautions to Prevent Transmission of Infectious Agents. [online] Available from: https://www.cdc.gov/infectioncontrol/pdf/guidelines/isolation-guidelines-H.pdf [Last accessed December, 2022].
28. Sims JR, Robinson NL, Moore EJ, Janus JR. Transoral robotic medial hypopharyngectomy: Surgical technique. Head Neck. 2016;38 Suppl 1: E2127-9.
29. Smith RV, Schiff BA, Sarta C, Hans S, Brasnu D. Transoral robotic total laryngectomy. Laryngoscope. 2013;123(3):678-82.
30. Tay JK, Khoo MLM, Loh WS. Surgical considerations for tracheostomy during the COVID-19 pandemic: lessons learned from the severe acute respiratory syndrome outbreak. JAMA Otolaryngol Head Neck Surg. 2020. 146(6):517-8.
31. Tsang RK, Holsinger FC. Transoral endoscopic nasopharyngectomy with a flexible next-generation robotic surgical system. Laryngoscope. 2016; 126(10):2257-62.
32. US Food and Drug Administration. (2009). 501 (k) Summary, Section III: Indications for Use for Intuitive Surgical Endoscopic Instrument Control System for Transoral Otolaryngology Procedures, 2009. [online] Available from: http://www.accessdata.fda.gov/cdrh_docs/pdf9/K090993.pdf [Last accessed December, 2022].
33. van Weert S, Rijken JA, Plantone F, Bloemena E, Vergeer MR, Lissenberg-Witte BI, et al. A systematic review on transoral robotic surgery (TORS) for carcinoma of unknown primary origin: Has tongue base mucosectomy become indispensable? Clin Otolaryngol. 2020;45(5):732-8.
34. Vianini M, Fiacchini G, Benettini G, Dallan I, Bruschini L. Experience in transoral robotic surgery in pediatric subjects: a systematic literature review. front surg. 2021;8:726739.
35. Vicini C, Dallan I, Canzi P, Frassineti S, La Pietra MG, Montevecchi F. Transoral robotic tongue base resection in obstructive sleep apnoea-hypopnoea syndrome: a preliminary report. ORL J Otorhinolaryngol Relat Spec. 2010;72(1):22-7.
36. Vicini C, Montevecchi F, Gobbi R, De Vito A, Meccariello G. Transoral robotic surgery for obstructive sleep apnea syndrome: Principles and technique. World J Otorhinolaryngol Head Neck Surg. 2017;3(2):97-100.
37. Weinstein GS, O'Malley BW Jr, Cohen MA, Quon H. Transoral robotic surgery for advanced oropharyngeal carcinoma. Arch Otolaryngol Head Neck Surg. 2010;136(11):1079-85.
38. Weinstein GS, O'Malley BW Jr, Hockstein NG. Transoral robotic surgery: supraglottic laryngectomy in a canine model. Laryngoscope. 2005;115(7): 1315-9.
39. Wei WI, Ho WK. Transoral robotic resection of recurrent nasopharyngeal carcinoma. Laryngoscope. 2010;120(10):2011-4.

40. Wei WI, Tuen HH, Ng RW, Lam LK. Safe tracheostomy for patients with severe acute respiratory syndrome. Laryngoscope. 2003;113(10):1777-9.
41. Wen CZ, Douglas JE, Elrakhawy M, Paul EA, Rassekh CH. Nuances and Management of Hilar Submandibular Sialoliths With Combined Transoral Robotic Surgery-Assisted Sialolithotomy and Sialendoscopy. Otolaryngol Head Neck Surg. 2021;165(1):76-82.
42. World Health Organisation. (2020). Rational use of personal protective equipment for coronavirus disease (COVID-19) and considerations during severe shortages. Interim Guidance. [online] Available from: https://www.who.int/publications/i/item/rational-use-of-personal-protective-equipment-for-coronavirus-disease-(covid-19)-and-considerations-during-severe-shortages [Last accessed December, 2022].

PIPAC: Technique and Applications in Gastrointestinal Oncology

CHAPTER 9

*Hugo Teixeira Farinha, Amaniel Kefleyesus,
Fabian Grass, Martin Hübner*

Abstract

Background: Current treatment modalities for patients with peritoneal carcinomatics cancer (PC) are limited and prognosis remains dismal. Pressurized Intraperitoneal aerosol chemotherapy (PIPAC) represents a minimally invasive treatment alternative with pharmacokinetic advantages. The present chapter aims to provide a comprehensive overview on practical aspects and clinical data reporting on feasibility, safety and efficacy.

Methods: Review of literature was done with regard to practical and surgical aspects. Review of experimental and clinical evidence of PIPAC with emphasis of PC from gastrointestinal (GI) origin.

Results: Laparoscopic access and repeatability rates were 83–100% and 32–82% with PC of various origins. For GI origin surgery-related complications were 0–9% and 0–12% for overall origin. In studies including GI origin, commonly described common terminology criteria for adverse events (CTCAE) grade 1–2 events were abdominal pain and nausea occurring in 10–33% of patients. CTCAE grades 3–5 were described in 0–30%. Procedure mortality rate was 1.6% for all PC origin. No hematological, renal or hepatic toxicity was observed even after repetitive administration. Median operation time of 98 minutes (IQR: 89–117) remained stable over time but is likely to decrease by adding electrostatic precipitation (ePIPAC). Quality-of-life and symptoms were not negatively impacted by repeated PIPAC. The treatment response according to RECIST was 44–77% and 45–91% according to peritoneal regression grading score (PRGS) in four phase II trials.

Conclusion: Standardization of the procedure and utilization of safety checklist allows safe introduction of PIPAC in clinical routine with minimal learning curve. Evidence from controlled trials and retrospective studies suggests that PIPAC is a feasible, safe, well-tolerated, and effective treatment option in patients with PC.

Keywords: PIPAC, peritoneal cancer, pressurized, intraperitoneal chemotherapy.

■ INTRODUCTION

Peritoneal carcinomatosis (PC) remains a diagnostic and therapeutic challenge with few available therapy options and a bad prognosis.[1-3] Outcomes are worse for PC compared to other advanced oncological situations, and response rates to systemic chemotherapy are poor with minimal tissue concentrations[4] due to poor peritoneal vascularization and limited tissue penetration.[5] Additionally, adverse effects are common, and as a result, the use of palliative chemotherapy has recently come under scrutiny.[6,7] Combining cytoreductive surgery (CRS) and hyperthermic intraperitoneal chemotherapy (HIPEC) appears to be effective and shows promising results (in whom curative surgery is feasible).[8] Nevertheless, the majority of patients with PC are not eligible for CRS and HIPEC because of the important morbi-mortality.[9,10]

It has been suggested that patients with advanced PC may benefit from the novel minimally invasive technique known as pressurized intraperitoneal aerosol chemotherapy (PIPAC). First human application took place in 2011 in Herne, Germany.[11-14] Pressured vaporization enables intraperitoneal administration of cytostatic agent with enhanced tissue penetration and distribution lead to greater concentrations despite lower cytostatic dosages.[15-17] Repetitive applications are permitted due to minimally invasive access without cytoreduction with reduction of the morbidity.[18,19] Two systematic reviews have been published with emphasis on clinical and experimental evidence.[20,21] Patients with PC from colorectal cancer have shown that PIPAC is possible, safe, and effective in retrospective and prospective clinical trials,[22] gastric cancer,[23] mesothelioma,[24] and ovarian cancer.[25] The aim of the present chapter was to highlight important practical aspects and to review the available scientific data on PIPAC with reference to its viability, safety, and effectiveness.

■ MATERIALS AND METHODS

All original scientific papers were considered to this chapter regarding practical and surgical aspects and experimental and clinical evidence of PIPAC including our institutional experience in Lausanne University Hospital (CHUV). Review articles and book chapters were not included. No language restrictions were applied. Results were analyzed and presented with special emphasis on GI tumors. This chapter does not include any research on intraperitoneal chemotherapy by conventional lavage (HIPEC) or by use of an intraperitoneal catheter (IPC).

■ RESULTS

Development of the Concept and Preclinical Data

Intraperitoneal application in a gaseous form of cytostatics under pressure was described in three studies, already in 1996.[15,16,26] A device to create a therapeutic pneumoperitoneum was first described in 2000,16 but technical limitations prevented clinical application at this point. A novel device with possibility for clinical application was designed in 2010 and first use in human was performed in November 2012.[13] The primary method of action of PIPAC as an intra-abdominal medication delivery system has been thoroughly investigated in preclinical studies. Biodistribution of molecules applied by PIPAC and conventional lavage (HIPEC model) was then tested in an ex vivo study.16 In the aerosolized specimen with aerosolization of drugs via a micropump, the test substance was found to have better distribution and tissue penetration than in the lavage model (HIPEC).[27,28] In tumor nodules, there was higher biological activity than in normal peritoneum up to a depth of 1 mm, but no activity was found after lavage.[12] Additionally, only the aerosol group received treatment on the anterior abdominal wall and hidden peritoneal surfaces.[29-32]

PIPAC Procedure Technique

Surgical technique was standardized by the pioneer group and described in detail by our group and others.[12,14,18,19] Pneumoperitoneum of 12 mm Hg carbon dioxide is made with the open implantation of two balloon trocars, one 10 mm and one 5 mm. Ascites is quantified, aspirated, and sent for cytology. Diagnostic laparoscopy included documentation of the extent of peritoneal carcinomatosis is done using the peritoneal cancer index (PCI).[33,34] Small biopsies of representative peritoneal nodules and peritonectomy of nondiseased area specimens were retrieved for pathological examination. Liquid chemotherapy is aerosolized by use of a pressure injector and a specific nebulizer (micropump). The micropump is attached to the pressure injector that is filled with liquid cytostatic solution and injected through a 10-mm trocar into the closed abdomen, which is confirmed by zero-flow CO_2. Cytostatic medications were created by clinical pharmacology following a medical oncologist's prescription and provided to the operating room as a liquid solution under tightly closed plastic covers **(Figs. 1 to 9)**.

For peritoneal carcinomatosis of colorectal origin, oxaliplatin at a dose of 92 mg/m^2 of body surface in 150 mL dextrose solution was suggested. According to the dose-finding trial, cisplatin (7.5 mg/m^2) and doxorubicin (1.5 mg/m^2) were initially used to treat peritoneal carcinomatosis of noncolorectal origin before being adjusted to 10.5 and 2.1 mg/m^2, respectively.[22,23,25] Cytostatics were applied at a flow rate of 30 mL/min for 30 minutes at a temperature of 37°C while being nebulized at the usual laparoscopic pressure of 12 mm Hg. After 30 minutes, the capnoperitoneum is evacuated with the use of a CAWS (Closed Aerosol Evacuation Waste System) equipped with two microparticle filters to capture residual molecules into the air waste system of the hospital. Contraindications to aerosols administration are inaccessible abdomen or bowel lesions during exploration. New methods adding electrostatic loading (ePIPAC) as an adjunct to aerosol

PIPAC: Technique and Applications in Gastrointestinal Oncology

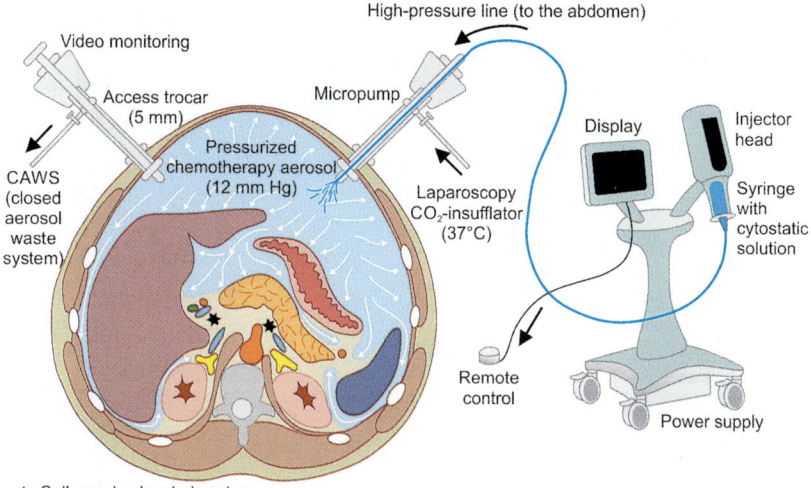

Fig. 1: Pressurized intraperitoneal aerosol chemotherapy (PIPAC). Two balloon trocars are used to access the abdomen. Using a specific nebulizer, liquid chemotherapy is administered as an aerosol.

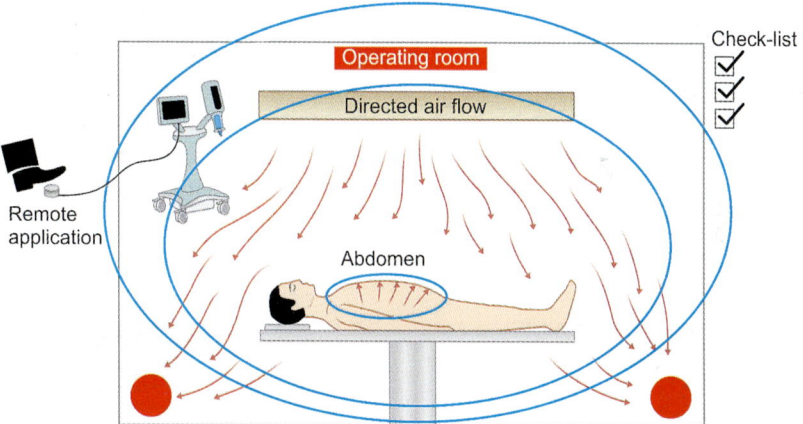

Fig. 2: Pressurized Intraperitoneal aerosol chemotherapy (PIPAC): Safety application. Leakage is prevented by three stages of containment:[11,19] (I) Balloon trocars and continual monitoring of the insufflator ensure an airtight capnoperitoneum. (II) Directed or laminar airflow. (III) Extending an aerosolized cytostatic treatment from outside the space. Only when all items on a predetermined checklist have been checked off pressurized intraperitoneal aerosol chemotherapy can only be applied if a standardized checklist is fully completed.[19]

and artificial hydrostatic pressure improved tissue uptake in a preclinical model. Furthermore, administration time could be reduced by 25 minutes.[28] PIPAC is administered repetitively (3 at least) at an interval of about 6 weeks. Safety protocol includes three levels of containment as recommended.[11] Before administering cytostatics, all parts of a dedicated safety checklist

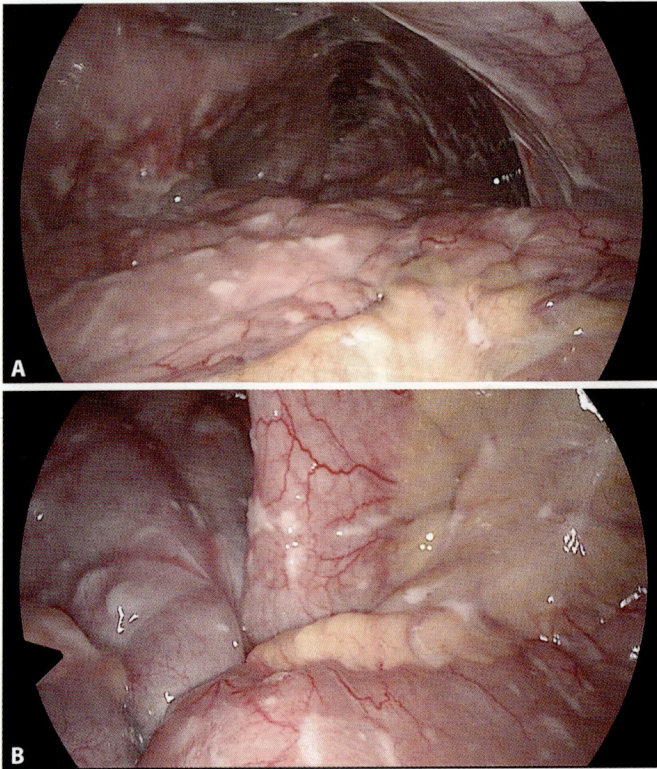

Figs. 3A and B: peritoneal carcinomatosis index (PCI) status documentation of a miliary peritoneal carcinosis (PCI-39) from gynecological origin. (A) Extensive dissemination in right upper and right flank areas; (B) Small bowel and colon with confluent implants.

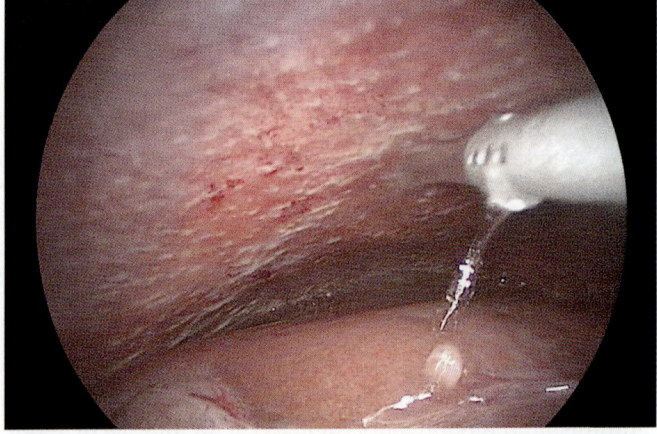

Fig. 4: Peritoneal washing cytology in right upper quadrant.

PIPAC: Technique and Applications in Gastrointestinal Oncology

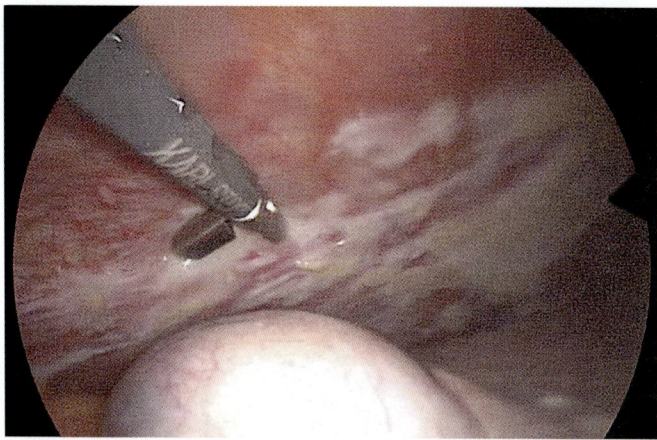

Fig. 5: Laparoscopic peritoneal biopsy of confluent implants from colorectal origin.

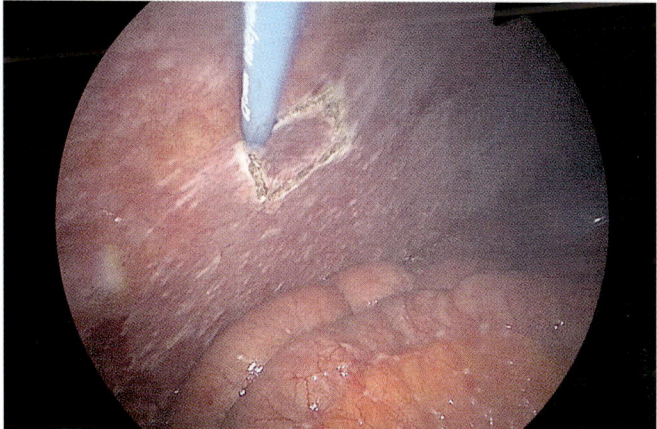

Fig. 6: Demarcation of the peritonectomy's edges with monopolar hook.

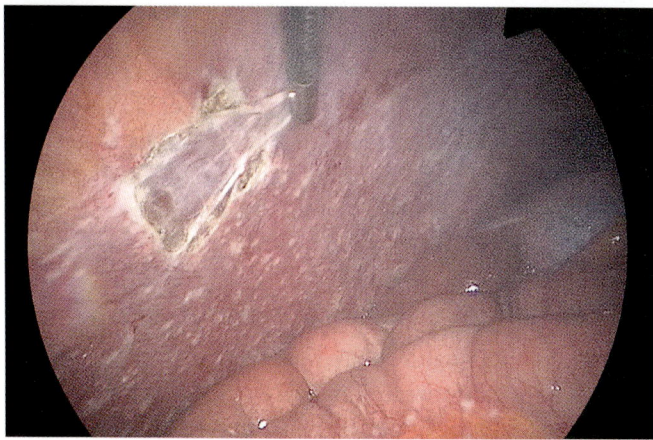

Fig. 7: Peritonectomy with biopsy forceps.

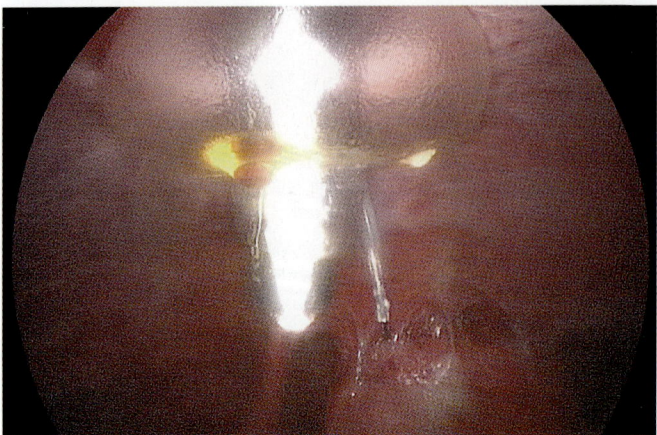

Fig. 8: Midline installation of the micro-pump and the electrode for electroprecipitation.

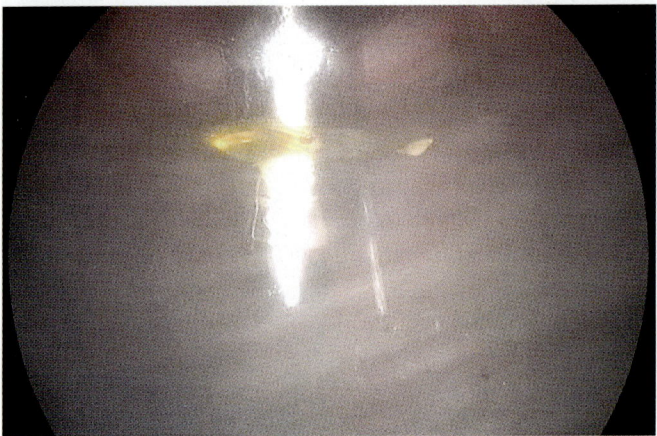

Fig. 9: Aerosolization of the chemotherapy through the micro-pump, with the so-called "snow storm".

(including staff and procedure-related safety aspects, team time out) are frequently double-checked. The original checklist from the German predecessor group served as the basis for actual checklist.[11] English version was also provided.[19] To promote adoption, standardize, and improve perioperative care in terms of nursing, drugs, blood tests, and nutrition, and a standardized clinical pathway (care map) can be employed.

Safety Strategy and Workplace Measurements

A rigorous occupational health safety policy was developed by the German precursor group.[11] Furthermore, because of environmental and safety aspects are of major relevance, these concerns have been widely studied.[11,19,35,36] Three different levels of confinement were suggested to rule out any risk for healthcare workers; laminar airflow and dilution capacity of the operating room; air-tight pneumoperitoneum (balloon trocars, zero flow); and remote application of cytostatics from outside the operating room (*see* **Fig. 2**). Air-pollution levels in actual clinical settings were measured.[36] Under actual PIPAC conditions, no cisplatin was detected in the air at the surgical team's and anesthesiologists' workstations (detection limit 0.000009 mg/m^3). Studies concluded that PIPAC did conform to the European Community working safety laws and regulations.

Implementation (Swiss experience)

PIPAC program was implemented at University Hospital of Lausanne, Switzerland (CHUV), in January 2015. A comparison was performed between PIPAC and other currently available alternatives. Resources, unknown, dangers and support were analyzed. PIPAC was judged as an interesting opportunity that appeared to be feasible with demonstrated benefits for selected cancer patients with PC. PIPAC was thus introduced at Lausanne University Hospital ingrained in an institutional review board approved research activity with support of the general hospital directional. Progressive or persistent PC during or after at least one course of systemic treatment qualified a patient for PIPAC treatment. In the absence of contraindications, potentially curative therapeutic options including cytoreductive surgery and HIPEC were always the preferred. Patients with symptomatic PC predominating and minimal disease elsewhere were given special consideration. The oncologist and surgeon saw each patient in an outpatient setting, and all indications were confirmed at the multidisciplinary tumor board. All patients gave written consent for PIPAC after receiving both oral and written information regarding the technique and complications of the treatment. Exclusion criteria for PIPAC were intestinal obstruction, thrombosis of the portal vein and contraindications to therapeutic capnoperitoneum. More than 35% of our patients had two or more laparotomies before PIPAC procedure.[18] All patients received palliative care because there are no long-term results from PIPAC treatment yet. All patients were specifically informed of this crucial issue during the preoperative information and consenting process. In line with current protocols, patients with PC of colorectal origin received oxaliplatin (92 mg/m^2), while a combination of cisplatin (7.5 mg/m^2) and doxorubicin (1.5 mg/m^2) was applied for the other malignancies.[19]

■ CLINICAL RESULTS

Feasibility and Safety

Clinical investigations show that in patients with PC of various origins, PIPAC was feasible, safe, and efficient.[20,21] The procedure was technically feasible in the large majority of patients with failure rate to access the abdomen (unsuccessful procedures/attempted procedures) between 0 and 17%. PIPAC treatment could be repeated in 32–82% of patients.[20,21] In an analysis of 15 studies including patients with PC from GI origin (colorectal, gastric, small bowel, and biliary tract), surgery-related complications were observed in 0–9% and 0–12% according to all clinical studies with PC from various origins.[14,18,22,23,25,36-49] Postoperative adverse events were assessed by the Common Terminology Criteria for Adverse Events (CTCAE) grading system in most studies.[50] In studies including GI origin, commonly described CTCAE grade 1–2 events included nausea and gastrointestinal pain, 33 and 10% respectively. CTCAE grades 3–5 were described in 0–37%. Only one clinical study report exclusively on PC of colorectal origin including 17 patients with toxicity grade CTCEA 3–5 of 23% and four study report exclusively on PC of gastric origin including 90 patients with toxicity grade CTCEA 3–5 of 20–37%. Including all clinical studies, mortality rate was 1.6%, with 37% of deceased patients deemed unrelated to the surgery, bringing the death risk associated with the procedure down to 1%. Mean hospital stay was 3 days.[20,21] In our experience, median operation time was overall 98 minutes (IQR: 89–117) with 91 minutes (IQR: 87–103), 93 minutes (IQR: 88–107), and 103 min (IQR: 91–121) for the first 20, 50, and 100 PIPAC, respectively.[19] Some clinical studies including PC from colorectal origin are displayed in **Table 1**.

In the Lausanne experience, there were no technical or safety difficulties that required abandoning an intervention.[19] All PIPAC procedures adhered to the safety checklist, which helped to prevent omissions in 9% of all interventions, such as missing protective eyewear, transparent protection sheets, cytostatic waste bins underneath injector heads, or CAWS that were not attached. In every instance, the checklist was satisfactorily finished before cytostatics were given. Minor incidents happened during nebulization in 11% of PIPAC operations. In 4% of PIPAC procedures, the high-pressure line's Y-connection needed to be repaired, but in all other cases, the leak was completely stopped by the clear coversheet that was placed over the pressure line. When doing a single-head injection, no leak was seen. In 7% of the cases, pressure limits (>200 PSI) was reached, resulting in an automated safety halt of injection. In all situations when the pressure restrictions were observed, application could be completed after a brief pause (1 minute). One PIPAC was delayed and completed after 15 minutes of charging time because the OR team forgot to charge the injector overnight.[19]

Toxicity and Systemic Uptake

Three studies evaluated organ-specific and systemic toxicity, as well as inflammatory response.[38,47,51] There was no significant systemic toxicity after PIPAC. Even after repetitive administration, no renal, hepatic or hematological toxicity was observed. Inflammatory response was throughout

TABLE 1: Clinical studies including patients with peritoneal cancer of gastrointestinal (GI) origin undergoing pressurized intraperitoneal aerosol chemotherapy (PIPAC).

Reference	Design	No. of patients (n)	Primary tumor	No. of PIPACs (n)	Access fail (%)	Histological response (%)	Toxicity (%CTCAE grades 1/2/3/4/5	Median overall survival (months)
Solass et al.[14]	Prospective case-series	3	• Gastric • Appendix • Ovarian	12	0	100 (2 complete 1 partial)	1/3/1/0/0	9
Odendahl et al.[40]	Observational, retrospective	91	• Gastric • Colorectal • Appendix • Ovarian • Mesothelioma	158	6	n/a	-/-/8/1/3	13.4
Demtröder et al.[22]	Retrospective	17	• Colorectal	48	13	Per protocol: 71–86	12/0/4/0/0	15.7
Nadiradze et al.[23]	Retrospective	25	• Gastric	60	8	Per protocol: 71	14/0/3/1/2	14.4
Robella et al.[38]	Retrospective	14	• Gastric • Colorectal • Appendix • Pseudomyxoma • Ovarian	40	2	n/a	6/8/0/0/0	n/a
Alyami et al.[49]	Retrospective	73	• Gastric • Colorectal • Pseudomyxoma • Ovarian	164	n/a	N/A	-/-/16/0/5	2.8

Contd...

Contd...

Reference	Design	No. of patients (n)	Primary tumor	No. of PIPACs (n)	Access fail (%)	Histological response (%)	Toxicity (%CTCAE grades 1/2/3/4/5)	Median overall survival (months)
Hübner et al.[18]	Retrospective	44	• Gastric • Colorectal • Ovarian	91	7	N/A	7/1/0/0/1	n/a
Falkenstein et al.[48]	Retrospective	13	Biliary tract	17	15	Per Protocol: 80	8/6/0/0/0	2.8
Giger-Pabst et al.[36]	Retrospective	512	• Gastric • Colorectal • Pseudomyxoma • Ovarian • Gynecologic • Mesothelioma	1,200	10	Per rotocol: 75	170/-/4/0/7	n/a
Nowacki et al.[46]	Retrospective/ International survey study	349	• Gastric • Colorectal • Ovarian	832	n/a	n/a	n/a	15.7
Teixeira et al.[54]	Retrospective	42	• Gastric • Colorectal • Small bowel • Ovarian • Mesothelioma	91	7	n/a	32/0/0/0/0	n/a

moderate and transient. Furthermore, the most recent cisplatin/doxorubicin dose escalation trial demonstrated no dose-limiting toxicities by Tempfer et al. using an intraperitoneal dose of 10.5 mg/m^2 and 2.1 mg/m^2, respectively.[42] Peripheral venous doxorubicin maximal concentrations after PIPAC were 4.0–6.2 ng/mL; half-lives ranged from 86 to 468 min.[14]

Efficacy

Long-term follow-up data are currently unavailable; in fact, the first human use was only described in November 2011.[11] The treatment response according to RECIST was 44–77% in four phase II trials, three of these including PC of GI origin had the same response[25,43,44,52-55] **(Table 2)**. Histological tumor regression rate for therapy-resistant PC assessed by consecutive samples taken during repetitive PIPAC was 62–100% including all clinical studies. Regarding the PC origin, histological regression was 62–88% for ovarian, 71–86% for colorectal and 70–100% for gastric origin but pathological assessment was inconsistent.[20] Consequently, a new peritoneal regression grading score (PRGS) was created to standardize histological evaluation.[53] According to PRGS, treatment response was 45–91% in phase II trials **(Table 2)**. Improvement of PCI for GI tumors has been demonstrated in only one clinical study in 64% of patients (47/73).[39] Median survival after PIPAC was 13.4–15.4 months for gastric and 15.7 months for colorectal peritoneal carcinomatosis.[20]

TABLE 2: Efficacy according to RECIST (Response evaluation criteria in solid tumors) criteria and peritoneal regression grading score (PRGS)[53] in Phase II studies including patients with peritoneal cancer of various origin undergoing Pressurized intraperitoneal aerosol chemotherapy (PIPAC).

Reference	Design	No. of patients (n)	Primary tumor	No. of PIPACs (n)	Access fail (%)	RECIST response (%)	PRGS response (%)
PIPAC-OV-1[25]	Phase II	64	Ovarian gynecologic	130	17	• ITT: 52 • PP: 62	• ITT: 62 • PP: 82
PIPAC-GA-1[43]	Phase II	25	Gastric	n/a	n/a	• ITT: 40 • PP: 77	• ITT: 36 • PP: 75
PIPAC-GA-2[55]	Phase II	31	Gastric	56	n/a	n/a	• ITT: N/A • PP: 92
PIPAC-OPC-1[44]	Phase II	35	• Gastric • Colorectal • Small bowel • Ovarian • Gyneco-logic	129	0	n/a	• ITT: 52 • PP: 67

(ITT: intention to treat; PP: per protocol)

Quality of Life

Quality-of-life (QoL) data during PIPAC was reported in eight studies.[24,25,38-40,44,45,54] QoL was determinate according to the SF-36 survey and EORTC-QLQ-30 questionnaire. In all studies, overall QoL was preserved during PIPAC. Improvement of global health was reported in two studies.[24,25] Functional measures of physical, emotional, cognitive, and social functioning improved in some studies while remaining stable in others.[24,25,40] In two studies, symptoms like nausea/vomiting, loss of appetite, constipation, and diarrhea decreased after PIPAC[24,25] and in the other experiments did not deteriorate. In five further studies, pain scores remained the same.[38,40,44]

■ DISCUSSION

Implementation of a new and potentially dangerous treatment as PIPAC can be difficult and complex. However, PIPAC could be safely introduced in clinical routine in several independent settings. Complete adherence to the established safety protocol and dedicated safety checklist remains mandatory in order to sustain PIPAC as standardized and safe procedure. As operation times and technological issues were minimal from the start and did not become worse with time, it is interesting to note that no learning curve was visible. This might be explained by how well-standardized PIPAC process is. Therefore, structured certification training must be completed before PIPAC is used as a novel treatment. Multidisciplinary collaboration is also mandatory. Creation of a dedicated individually trained surgical and medical oncology team together with repetitive information and training to all actors involved in the PIPAC program are an additional safety factor. Nowadays PIPAC has been accepted as emerging and promising treatment option. Active treatment facilities follow a well-established PIPAC therapy protocol, and consistent outcomes and treatment effects have been observed.[46]

The majority of patients with resistant peritoneal carcinomatosis of GI or other sources were found to be amenable to this innovative technique. Low rates of postoperative morbidity and intraoperative complications were observed. PIPAC was followed by a moderate and transient inflammatory response that was proportionate to the disease burden. Neither renal hepatic nor hematological toxicity was noticed even after repetitive procedures. Short-term oncological outcomes are encouraging but actual data are limited by absence of control groups, small sample size, and heterogeneity.

Quality-of-life and symptoms were not impacted by PIPAC treatment. This is an important aspect as long as PIPAC is a palliative therapy. Evidently, PIPAC does not have major systemic side effects like systemic chemotherapy does. In no PIPAC study were neurotoxicity, myelotoxicity, alopecia, or fatigue observed, which are common with subsequent courses of systemic chemotherapy and worsen QoL.

Preliminary favorable response rates ask for more prospective analysis regarding oncological efficacy. There are numerous ongoing clinical trials for peritoneal carcinomatosis patients undergoing PIPAC. Audit of performance and outcomes is integral part of critical evaluation of a new treatment and publication of results makes for transparency and credibility. Algorithms with previously chosen indications and contraindications to the readily available treatment options (HIPEC, PIPAC, and systemic chemotherapy) are also necessary. To facilitate study comparison, future research should identify consistent endpoints, and comparative groups are crucial to strengthen the body of evidence. Comparative research on individuals with advanced cancer, however, may provide an ethical and methodological challenge.

■ CONCLUSION

Current treatment modalities for patients with peritoneal cancer are limited and the prognosis remains poor. Pressurized intraperitoneal aerosol chemotherapy (PIPAC)represents a minimally invasive treatment alternative with pharmacokinetic advantages. The standardization of the procedure and the use of the safety checklist allow a safe introduction of PIPAC into clinical routine with a minimal learning curve. Evidence from controlled trials and retrospective studies suggests that PIPAC is a feasible, safe, well-tolerated treatment option. The first preliminary clinical results are promising in patients with isolated peritoneal disease.

Sources of support and funding for this work: None.

■ REFERENCES

1. Bloemendaal ALA, Verwaal VJ, van Ruth S, Boot H, Zoetmulder FAN. Conventional surgery and systemic chemotherapy for peritoneal carcinomatosis of colorectal origin: A prospective study. Eur J Surg Oncol. 2005;31(10):1145-51.
2. Jayne DG, Fook S, Loi C, Seow-Choen F. Peritoneal carcinomatosis from colorectal cancer. Br J Surg. 2002;89(12):1545-50.
3. Sadeghi B, Arvieux C, Glehen O, Beaujard AC, Rivoire M, Baulieux J, et al. Peritoneal carcinomatosis from non-gynecologic malignancies: Results of the EVOCAPE 1 multicentric prospective study. Cancer. 2000;88(2):358-63.
4. Dedrick RL, Flessner MF. Pharmacokinetic problems in peritoneal drug administration: Tissue penetration and surface exposure. J Natl Cancer Inst. 1997;89(7):480-7..
5. Markman M. Intraperitoneal antineoplastic drug delivery: rationale and results. Lancet Oncol. 2003;4(5):277-83.
6. Sun CC, Frumovitz M, Bodurka DC. Quality of life and gynecologic malignancies. Curr Oncol Rep. 2005;7(6):459-65.
7. Kayl AE, Meyers CA. Side-effects of chemotherapy and quality of life in ovarian and breast cancer patients. Curr Opin Obstet Gynecol. 2006;18(1):24-8..
8. Glehen O, Gilly FN, Boutitie F, Bereder JM, Quenet F, Sideris L, et al. Toward curative treatment of peritoneal carcinomatosis from nonovarian origin

by cytoreductive surgery combined with perioperative intraperitoneal chemotherapy: A multi-institutional study of 1290 patients. Cancer. 2010; 116(24):5608-18.
9. Verwaal VJ. Long-term results of cytoreduction and HIPEC followed by systemic chemotherapy. Cancer J. 2009;15(3):212-5.
10. Verwaal VJ, van Ruth S, de Bree E, van Slooten GW, van Tinteren H, Boot H, et al. Randomized trial of cytoreduction and hyperthermic intraperitoneal chemotherapy versus systemic chemotherapy and palliative surgery in patients with peritoneal carcinomatosis of colorectal cancer. J Clin Oncol. 2003;21(20):3737-43.
11. Solass W, Giger-Pabst U, Zieren J, Reymond MA. Pressurized intraperitoneal aerosol chemotherapy (PIPAC): occupational health and safety aspects. Ann Surg Oncol. 2013;20(11):3504-11.
12. Solass W, Herbette A, Schwarz T, Hetzel A, Sun JS, Dutreix M, et al. Therapeutic approach of human peritoneal carcinomatosis with Dbait in combination with capnoperitoneum: Proof of concept. Surg Endosc. 2012;26(3):847-52.
13. Solaß W, Hetzel A, Nadiradze G, Sagynaliev E, Reymond MA. Description of a novel approach for intraperitoneal drug delivery and the related device. Surg Endosc. 2012;26(7):1849-55.
14. Solass W, Kerb R, Mürdter T, Giger-Pabst U, Strumberg D, Tempfer C, et al. Intraperitoneal chemotherapy of peritoneal carcinomatosis using pressurized aerosol as an alternative to liquid solution: First evidence for efficacy. Ann Surg Oncol. 2014;21(2):553-9.
15. Esquis P, Consolo D, Magnin G, Pointaire P, Moretto P, Ynsa MD, et al. High intra-abdominal pressure enhances the penetration and antitumor effect of intraperitoneal cisplatin on experimental peritoneal carcinomatosis. Ann Surg. 2006;244(1):106-12.
16. Facy O, Al Samman S, Magnin G, Ghiringhelli F, Ladoire S, Chauffert B, et al. High pressure enhances the effect of hyperthermia in intraperitoneal chemotherapy with oxaliplatin: An experimental study. Ann Surg. 2012;256(6):1084-8.
17. Minchinton AI, Tannock IF. Drug penetration in solid tumours. Nat Rev Cancer. 2006;6(8):583-92.
18. Hübner M, Teixeira Farinha H, Grass F, Wolfer A, Mathevet P, Hahnloser D, et al. Feasibility and Safety of Pressurized Intraperitoneal Aerosol Chemotherapy for Peritoneal Carcinomatosis: A Retrospective Cohort Study. Gastroenterol Res Pract. 2017;2017:6852749.
19. Hübner M, Grass F, Teixeira-Farinha H, Pache B, Mathevet P, Demartines N. Pressurized IntraPeritoneal Aerosol Chemotherapy – Practical aspects. Eur J Surg Oncol. 2017;43(6):1102-9.
20. Grass F, Vuagniaux A, Teixeira-Farinha H, Lehmann K, Demartines N, Hübner M. Systematic review of pressurized intraperitoneal aerosol chemotherapy for the treatment of advanced peritoneal carcinomatosis. Br J Surg. 2017;104(6):669-78.
21. Tempfer C, Giger-Pabst U, Hilal Z, Dogan A, Rezniczek GA. Pressurized intraperitoneal aerosol chemotherapy (PIPAC) for peritoneal carcinomatosis: systematic review of clinical and experimental evidence with special emphasis on ovarian cancer. Archives of Gynecology and Obstetrics. 2018;298(2):243-57.
22. Demtröder C, Solass W, Zieren J, Strumberg D, Giger-Pabst U, Reymond MA. Pressurized intraperitoneal aerosol chemotherapy with oxaliplatin in colorectal peritoneal metastasis. Color Dis. 2016;18(4):364-71.

23. Nadiradze G, Giger-Pabst U, Zieren J, Strumberg D, Solass W, Reymond MA. Pressurized Intraperitoneal Aerosol Chemotherapy (PIPAC) with Low-Dose Cisplatin and Doxorubicin in Gastric Peritoneal Metastasis. J Gastrointest Surg. 2016;20(2):367-73.
24. Giger-Pabst U, Demtröder C, Falkenstein TA, Ouaissi M, Götze TO, Rezniczek GA, et al. Pressurized IntraPeritoneal Aerosol Chemotherapy (PIPAC) for the treatment of malignant mesothelioma. BMC Cancer. 2018;18(1):442.
25. Tempfer CB, Winnekendonk G, Solass W, Horvat R, Giger-Pabst U, Zieren J, et al. Pressurized intraperitoneal aerosol chemotherapy in women with recurrent ovarian cancer: A phase 2 study. Gynecol Oncol. 2015;137(2):223-8.
26. Jacquet P, Stuart OA, Chang D, Sugarbaker PH. Effects of intra-abdominal pressure on pharmacokinetics and tissue distribution of doxorubicin after intraperitoneal administration. Anticancer Drugs. 1996;7(5):596-603.
27. Jung DH, Son SY, Oo AM, Park YS, Shin DJ, Ahn SH, et al. Feasibility of hyperthermic pressurized intraperitoneal aerosol chemotherapy in a porcine model. Surg Endosc. 2016;30(10):4258-64.
28. Kakchekeeva T, Demtröder C, Herath NI, Griffiths D, Torkington J, Solaß W, et al. In Vivo Feasibility of Electrostatic Precipitation as an Adjunct to Pressurized Intraperitoneal Aerosol Chemotherapy (ePIPAC). Ann Surg Oncol. 2016;23(Suppl 5):592-8.
29. Khosrawipour V, Bellendorf A, Khosrawipour C, Hedayat-Pour Y, Diaz-Carballo D, Förster E, et al. Irradiation does not increase the penetration depth of doxorubicin in normal tissue after pressurized intra-peritoneal aerosol chemotherapy (PIPAC) in an ex vivo model. In Vivo (Brooklyn). 2016; 2016;30(5):593-7.
30. Khosrawipour V, Khosrawipour T, Kern AJP, Osma A, Kabakci B, Diaz-Carballo D, et al. Distribution pattern and penetration depth of doxorubicin after pressurized intraperitoneal aerosol chemotherapy (PIPAC) in a postmortem swine model. J Cancer Res Clin Oncol. 2016;142(11):2275-80.
31. Khosrawipour V, Khosrawipour T, Diaz-Carballo D, Förster E, Zieren J, Giger-Pabst U. Exploring the Spatial Drug Distribution Pattern of Pressurized Intraperitoneal Aerosol Chemotherapy (PIPAC). Ann Surg Oncol. 2016;23(4):1220-4.
32. Khosrawipour V, Khosrawipour T, Falkenstein Ta, Diaz-Carballo D, Förster E, Osma A, et al. Evaluating the Effect of Micropump© Position, Internal Pressure and Doxorubicin Dosage on Efficacy of Pressurized Intraperitoneal Aerosol Chemotherapy (PIPAC) in an Ex Vivo Model. Anticancer Res. 2016; 36(9):4595-600.
33. Portilla AG, Shigeki K, Baratti D, Deraco M. The intraoperative staging systems in the management of peritoneal surface malignancy. J Surg Oncol. 2008;98(4):228-31.
34. da Silva RG, Sugarbaker PH. Analysis of Prognostic factors in seventy patients having a complete cytoreduction plus Perioperative Intraperitoneal Chemotherapy for Carcinomatosis from Colorectal Cancer. J Am Coll Surg. 2006;203(6):878-86.
35. Oyais A, Solass W, Zieren J, Reymond MA, Giger-Pabst U. Occupational Health Aspects of Pressurised Intraperitoneal Aerosol Chemotherapy (PIPAC): Confirmation of Harmlessness. Zentralbl Chir. 2016;141(4):421-4.

36. Giger-Pabst U, Tempfer CB. How to Perform Safe and Technically Optimized Pressurized Intraperitoneal Aerosol Chemotherapy (PIPAC): Experience After a Consecutive Series of 1200 Procedures. J Gastrointest Surg. 2018; 2018;22(12): 2187-93.
37. Graversen M, Detlefsen S, Bjerregaard JK, Pfeiffer P, Mortensen MB. Peritoneal metastasis from pancreatic cancer treated with pressurized intraperitoneal aerosol chemotherapy (PIPAC). Clin Exp Metastasis. 2018;35(7):635-40.
38. Robella M, Vaira M, De Simone M. Safety and feasibility of pressurized intraperitoneal aerosol chemotherapy (PIPAC) associated with systemic chemotherapy: an innovative approach to treat peritoneal carcinomatosis. World J Surg Oncol. 2016;14:128.
39. Tempfer CB, Rezniczek GA, Ende P, Solaß W, Reymond MA, Solass W, et al. Pressurized Intraperitoneal Aerosol Chemotherapy with Cisplatin and Doxorubicin in Women with Peritoneal Carcinomatosis: A Cohort Study. Anticancer Res. 2015;35(12):6723-9.
40. Odendahl K, Solass W, Demtröder C, Giger-Pabst U, Zieren J, Tempfer C, et al. Quality of life of patients with end-stage peritoneal metastasis treated with Pressurized Intraperitoneal Aerosol Chemotherapy (PIPAC). Eur J Surg Oncol. 2015;41(10):1379-85.
41. Tempfer CB, Celik I, Solass W, Buerkle B, Pabst UG, Zieren J, et al. Activity of Pressurized Intraperitoneal Aerosol Chemotherapy (PIPAC) with cisplatin and doxorubicin in women with recurrent, platinum-resistant ovarian cancer: Preliminary clinical experience. Gynecol Oncol. 2014;132(2):307-11.
42. Tempfer CB, Giger-Pabst U, Seebacher V, Petersen M, Dogan A, Rezniczek GA. A phase I, single-arm, open-label, dose escalation study of intraperitoneal cisplatin and doxorubicin in patients with recurrent ovarian cancer and peritoneal carcinomatosis. Gynecol Oncol. 2018;150(1):23-30.
43. Struller F, Horvath P, Solass W, Weinreich FJ, Konigsrainer A, Reymond MA. Pressurized intraperitoneal aerosol chemotherapy with low-dose cisplatin and doxorubicin (PIPAC C/D) in patients with gastric cancer and peritoneal metastasis (PIPAC-GA1). J Clin Oncol. 2017.
44. Graversen M, Detlefsen S, Bjerregaard JK, Fristrup CW, Pfeiffer P, Mortensen MB. Prospective, single-center implementation and response evaluation of pressurized intraperitoneal aerosol chemotherapy (PIPAC) for peritoneal metastasis. Ther Adv Med Oncol. 2018;10:1758835918777036.
45. Robella M, Vaira M BA et al. Feasibility, efficacy, and safety of PIPAC with oxaliplatin, cisplatin, and doxorubicin in patients with peritoneal carcinomatosis from colorectal, ovarian, gastric cancers, and primary cancers of the peritoneum: an open-label, single-arm, phase II clin. In: Jacksonville FL (Ed). International symposium on regional cancer therapies of the society of surgical oncology; Chicago, Illinois: society of Surgical Oncology; 2018.
46. Nowacki M, Alyami M, Villeneuve L, Mercier F, Hubner M, Willaert W, et al. Multicenter comprehensive methodological and technical analysis of 832 pressurized intraperitoneal aerosol chemotherapy (PIPAC) interventions performed in 349 patients for peritoneal carcinomatosis treatment: an international survey study. Eur J Surg Oncol. 2018;44(7):991-6.
47. Farinha HT, Grass F, Labgaa I, Pache B, Demartnes N, Hübner M. Inflammatory response and toxicity after Pressurized Intraperitoneal Aerosol Chemotherapy. J Cancer. 2018;9(1):13-20

48. Falkenstein TA, Götze TO, Ouaissi M, Tempfer CB, Giger-Pabst U, Demtröder C. First clinical data of pressurized intraperitoneal aerosol chemotherapy (PIPAC) as salvage therapy for peritoneal metastatic biliary tract cancer. Anticancer Res. 2018;38(1):373-8.
49. Alyami M, Gagniere J, Sgarbura O, Cabelguenne D, Villeneuve L, Pezet D, et al. Multicentric initial experience with the use of the pressurized intraperitoneal aerosol chemotherapy (PIPAC) in the management of unresectable peritoneal carcinomatosis. Eur J Surg Oncol. 2017;43(11):2178-83.
50. National Cancer Institute. Common Terminology Criteria for Adverse Events (CTCAE). United States: National Institutes of Health Publication; 2009.
51. Blanco A, Giger-Pabst U, Solass W, Zieren J, Reymond MA. Renal and hepatic toxicities after pressurized intraperitoneal aerosol chemotherapy (PIPAC). Ann Surg Oncol. 2013;20(7):2311-6.
52. Robella M, Vaira M, De Simone M, Graversen M, Detlefsen S, Bjerregaard JK, et al. Prospective, single-center implementation and response evaluation of pressurized intraperitoneal aerosol chemotherapy (PIPAC) for peritoneal metastasis. Gynecol Oncol. 2018;10:1758835918777036.
53. Wiebke Solass, Christine Sempoux, Sönke Detlefsen NJC and FB. Peritoneal sampling and histological assessment of therapeutic response in peritoneal metastasis: proposal of the Peritoneal Regression Grading Score (PRGS). Pleura and Peritoneum. 2016;1(2):99-107.
54. Teixeira Farinha H, Grass F, Kefleyesus A et al. Impact of pressurized intraperitoneal aerosol chemotherapy on quality of life and symptoms in patients with peritoneal carcinomatosis: a retrospective cohort study. Gastroenterol Res Pract. 2017;2017:4596176.
55. Khomiakov V, Ryabov A, Bolotina LV et al. Bidirectional chemotherapy in gastric cancer (GC) with peritoneal carcinomatosis (PC) combining intravenous chemotherapy with intraperitoneal chemotherapy with low-dose cisplatin and doxorubicin administered as a pressurized aerosol: An open-label, phase II study. Pleura Peritoneum. 2016;1(3):159-166.

CHAPTER 10

Robotic Bariatric Surgery

Arun Prasad

■ INTRODUCTION

Robotic surgery has become more and more popular and acceptable to surgeons and medical fraternity at large in the last few years. The 3D vision and control of four ports have made a tremendous difference for dissection of delicate and friable structures. There is advantage of articulating instruments for suturing in small remote spaces as the instruments can do wrist-like movements. That has shown to improve the performance of intracorporeal suturing and also made it a safer option.[1]

Urology procedures were the areas that initially benefitted from robotic surgery.[2] The popularity in general and gastrointestinal (GI) surgery came late due to the initial misconception that this technology is best suited for one quadrant of the abdomen at a time.[3]

Roux-en-Y gastric bypass surgery is one of the most common bariatric surgery and is technically challenging compared to banding and sleeve surgeries. During robotic surgery, initially a hybrid method was adopted whereby the roux loop and small bowel manipulation was done by laparoscopy and robotic surgery was used for the more complex gastrojejunostomy anastomosis.[4] Dual-docking techniques were also followed where the robot is docked twice, once for infracolic compartment surgery followed by the supracolic compartment surgery. This was earliest reported in 2005 by Mohr et al.[5]

First robotic sleeve gastrectomy was reported in 2011 by Ayloo et al.[6]

First robotic mini gastric bypass-one anastomosis gastric bypass (MGB-OAGB) was done by Prasad in 2012.[7] It was also followed up at other centers in India, USA, and Turkey. MGB-OAGB is getting rapidly popular and is now considered worldwide as a good alternative to the Roux-en-Y bypass.[8-10] This procedure is also possible without the need of hybrid or dual docking.

Various studies comparing robotic and laparoscopic bariatric surgeries show no significant differences as far as surgery time, length of hospital stay, complications, or rate of conversion to open surgery is concerned,[10-12] but incidence of the postoperative anastomotic leaks, strictures, and bleeding have been shown to be significantly less in the robot-assisted surgery.[13]

The main advantages of robotic surgery are the 3D imaging, tremor filter, and articulated instruments that compensate some of the limitations of laparoscopic surgery such as restrictions in the range of motion of the instruments, and the poor ergonomic positioning that the surgeon feels during advanced procedures.[14] This is a new and evolving procedure and there is tremendous scope for improvement.

■ ADVANTAGES

The main advantages of robotic bariatric surgery can be listed as:
- 3D vision which is truly binocular
- Motion scaling of complex movements
- Wrist articulation leading to a 360° movement
- Fluid movement of instruments
- Tremor filter
- Remote sensing technology with the robotic staplers
- Ergonomically intuitive
- 25X magnification
- Teleproctoring possibilities
- Less head-up tilt of the table needed
- Lesser abdominal wall pressures needed as the robotic cannulas lift the abdominal wall
- Less torque to abdominal wall due to the instrument movements at fulcrum level
- Articulated instruments help in dissection at angles **(Figs. 1 and 2)**
- Ease of sutured anastomosis.

■ DISADVANTAGES
- High setting-up costs
- Expensive consumables

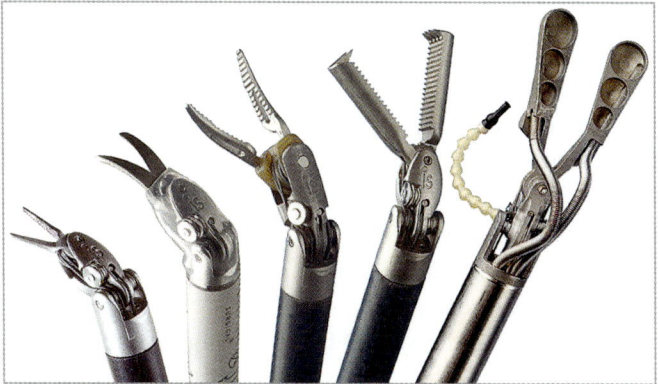

Fig. 1: Articulating instruments.

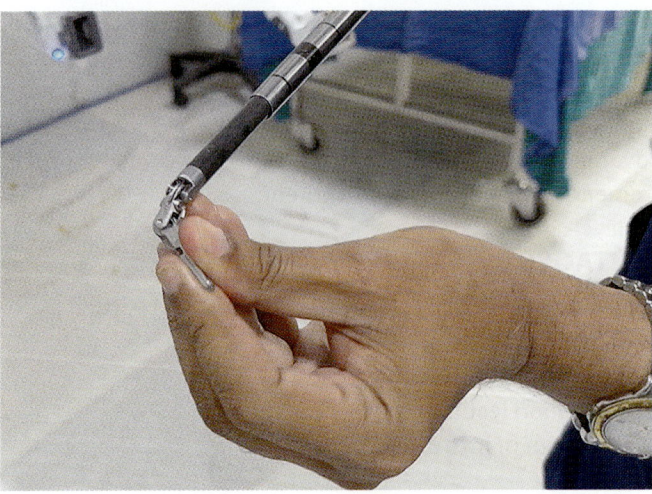

Fig. 2: Articulating instrument.

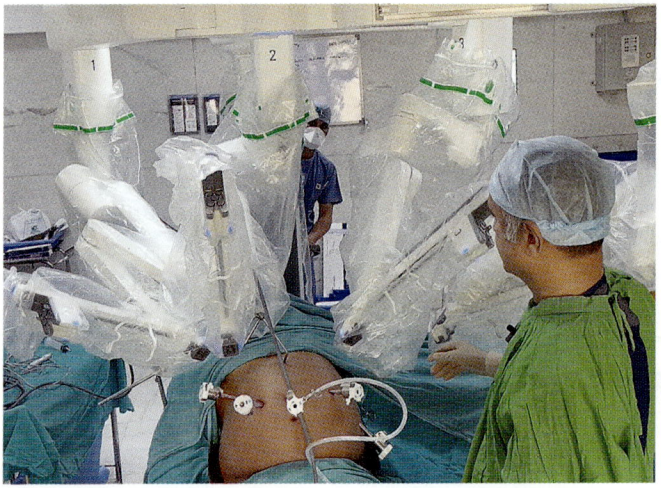

Fig. 3: Docking.

- Limited centers only
- Lack of tactile feedback
- Bulky apparatus occupying space
- Need for special training.

■ PROCEDURE DETAILS

Robot is docked from the head end of the patient or from one of the shoulder levels depending on surgeon preference **(Fig. 3)**.

Port positions are as shown in **Figure 4**. Epigastrium is used to insert a Nathanson retractor. Telescope is placed in the port about 5–10 cm supraumbilically depending upon patient's built. One port is introduced

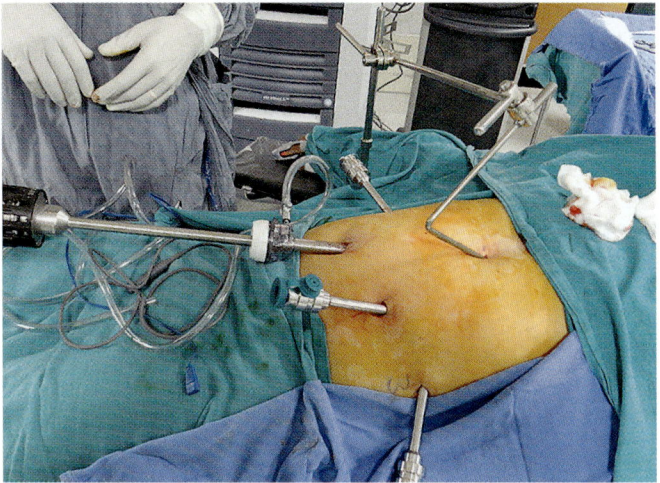

Fig. 4: Port positions.

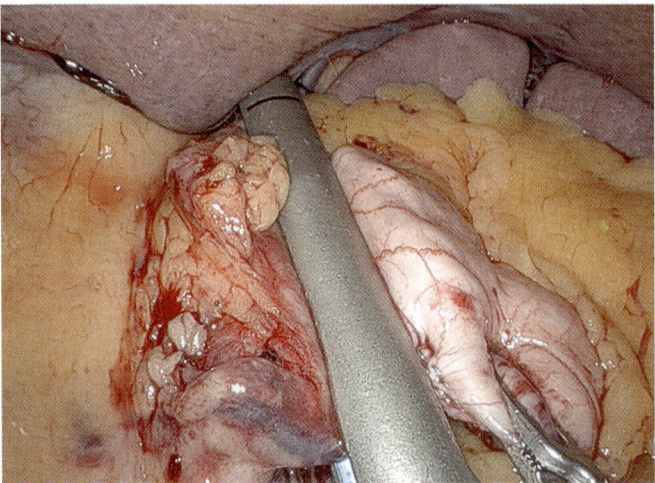

Fig. 5: Robotic stapler.

in the mid-clavicular line about 5 cm below the subcostal margins. One assistant port is introduced at the level of the camera port, laterally in the anterior axillary line. Stapler port of 12 mm is introduced 5 cm below and lateral to the right hypochondrial port.

Surgery usually is carried out using an energy device (harmonic or vessel sealer), bipolar grasper, atraumatic grasper, and a needle holder. The fifth port is used by assistant to use suction, scissors, suture introduction, etc.

Steps of the procedure is like laparoscopic bariatric procedures. Staplers can be robotic **(Fig. 5)** or regular laparoscopic by assistant. Sutured anastomosis **(Fig. 6)** are usually preferred as they have lower bleed, stricture, and leak rates.

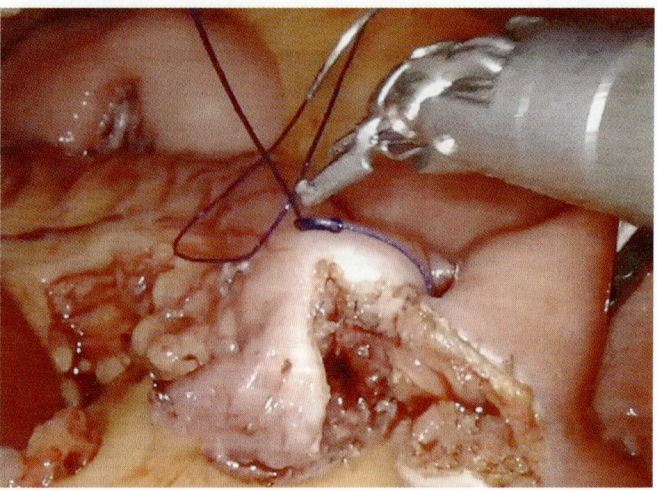

Fig. 6: Suturing.

■ COMPLICATIONS

Specific complications related to robotic surgery are as follows:
- Traction injury to viscera if there is uncoordinated movement
- Breaking of sutures while tightening due to lack of tactile feedback
- Bleeding due to accidental movement by surgeon or assistant. Complications stated above are unlikely after the initial learning curve.

■ TRAINING

There are training centers set up by various robotic companies. They also arrange for observership and proctorship for new trainees. Conferences and live workshops help in getting tips and discussing problems. Dual console and tele proctorship are special advantages with this technology.

■ DISCUSSION

Amongst all the advanced laparoscopic surgical procedures, bariatric surgery is extremely challenging due to the obese abdomen. It leads to torque both on the muscles of the patient and surgeon. There is intracorporeal resection and anastomosis of stomach and intestines. Tissue dissection, telescope and instrument handling can be difficult too.[15]

Robotic surgery has helped overcome some of these challenges to make the surgery technically less demanding and safer. Steady control of the telescope by the robotic arm is superior to assistant holding it.[16] Also, robotic suturing is more accurate and faster for GI anastomosis compared to its laparoscopic counterpart. Oblique and angulated anastomosis are less demanding by robotic surgery.[17] So is the tissue manipulation and alignment.[18]

After the learning curve, the time taken for the procedure is same for robotic and laparoscopic surgery. The added benefits of robotic surgery is seen both for the surgeon and the patient.

■ CONCLUSION

Technical challenges faced by surgeons during advanced laparoscopic surgeries have been reduced by a considerable extent by the advent of robotic surgery. Surgery in the obese, especially when dealing with super obese or situations of revision bariatric surgery, has been simplified by the robotic option. This is mainly true during the dissection behind the stomach, sutured gastrojejunostomy, and mesentery closure.

Robotic surgery is not here to replace laparoscopic surgery, but should be considered as an added tool in the armamentarium of surgeons when tackling difficult surgical situations.

■ REFERENCES

1. Stefanidis D, Wanf F, Korndorffer JR, Dunne JB, Scott DJ. Robotic assistance improves intracorporeal suturing performance and safety in the operating room while decreasing operator workload. Surg Endosc. 2010;24:377-82.
2. Menon M, Shrivastava A, Tewari A, Sarle R, Hemal A, Peabody JO, et al. Laparoscopic and robot assisted radical prostatectomy: establishment of a structured program and preliminary analysis of outcomes. J Urol. 2002;168:945-9.
3. Jacobsen G, Berger R, Horgan S. The role of robotic surgery in morbid obesity. J Laparoendosc Adv Surg Tech. 2003;13:279-83.
4. Ayloo SM, Addeo P, Shah G, Sbrana F, Giulianotti PC. Robot-assisted Hybrid Laparoscopic Roux-en-Y Gastric Bypass: Surgical Technique and Early Outcomes. J Laparoendosc Adv Surg Tech A. 2010;20(10):847-50.
5. Mohr C, Nadzam G, Curet M. Totally robotic Roux-en-Y gastric bypass. Arch Surg. 2005;140:779-85.
6. Ayloo S, Buchs N, Addeo P, Bianco FM, Giulanotti PC. Robot-assisted sleeve gastrectomy for super-morbidly obese patients. J Laproendosc Advan Surg Tech. 2011;21:295-9.
7. Prasad A. Robotic one anastomosis (omega loop/mini) gastric bypass for morbid obesity. J Robotic Surg. 2014;8:371-4.
8. Rutledge R. The Mini-Gastric Bypass: Experience with the First 1,274 Cases. Obes Surg. 2001;11:276-80.
9. Lee WJ, Ser KH, Lee YC, Tsou JJ, Chen SC, Chen JC. Laparoscopic Roux-en-Y vs mini-gastric bypass for the treatment of morbid obesity: a 10-year experience. Obes Surg. 20122;2:1827-34.
10. Musella M, Susa A, Greco F, De Luca M, Manno E, Di Stefano C, et al. The laparoscopic mini-gastric bypass: the Italian experience: outcomes from 974 consecutive cases in a multicenter review. Surg Endosc. 2014;28(1):156-63.
11. Allemann P, Leroy J, Asakuma M, Al Abeidi F, Dallemagne B, Marescaux J. Robotics may overcome technical limitations of single-trocar surgery. Arch Surg. 2010;145:267-71.

12. Maeso S, Resa M, Mayol JA, Blasco JA, Guerra M, Andradas E, et al. Efficacy of the Da Vinci surgical system in abdominal surgery compare with that of laparoscopy. Ann Surg. 2010;252(2):254-62.
13. Frazzoni M, Conigliaro R, Colli G, Melotti G. Conventional versus robot-assisted laparoscopic Nissen fundoplication: a comparison of postoperative acid reflux parameters. Surg Endosc. 2012;26:1675-81.
14. Tieu K1, Allison N, Snyder B, Wilson T, Toder M, Wilson E. Robotic-assisted Roux-en-Y gastric bypass: update from 2 high-volume centers. Surg Obes Relat Dis. 2013;9(2):284-8.
15. Macedo AL de V, Marcondes W, Junior BT, Steinwurz F. Secrets for successful laparoscopic antireflux surgery: robotic surgery. Ann Lap Endo Surg. 2017; 2(67):1-4.
16. Omote K, Feussner H, Ungeheuer A. Self-guided robotic camera control for laparoscopic surgery compared with human camera control. Am J Surg. 1999; 177:321-4.
17. Ruurda JP, Broeders AMJ, Pulles B, Kappelhof FM, van der Werken C. Manual robot assisted endoscopic suturing: time-action analysis in an experimental model. Surg Endosc. 2004;18:1249-52.
18. Talamini MA, Chapman S, Horgan S, Melvin WS. The Academic Robotics Group, A prospective analysis of 211 robotic-assisted surgical procedures. Surg Endosc. 2003;17:1521-4.

CHAPTER 11
Robot-assisted Liver Resection

Gursev Sandlas

■ INTRODUCTION

Minimally invasive surgery in children has grown by leaps and bounds over the last three decades mimicking the curve taken by the adult minimally invasive surgery.

Robot-assisted surgery has also grown in consonance with its adult counterpart with majority of the growth and innovation being driven by the pediatric urologists, to an extent that pyeloplasty and ureteric reimplantation have become the commonly performed robot-assisted procedures in children.[1]

Minimally invasive liver resection (MILR) however continues to be among the last bastions that need to be conquered both in adults as well as in children.

Minimally invasive liver resection in children suffers from paucity of published literature. Apart from sporadic case reports[2] and small series, there is definite lack of hard evidence when it comes to MILR. Though the obvious advantages of the minimally invasive approach in the form of reduced pain, early recovery and early commencement of activity remain unchallenged; overall outcomes though claimed to be same as open surgeries need further volumes to validate.

Robot-assisted hepatobiliary surgery in the form of surgery for choledochal cyst and biliary atresia is well documented with several large series published on the same. There is a complete paucity of literature on robot-assisted liver resections.[3,4]

Thus far, even laparoscopic hepatectomies that are reported in children are case reports and small case series of nonanatomical resections for small, peripheral, and isolated lesions[5-10] except one series.[11] Hence, the obvious advantages of robotic surgery which are so clearly elucidated with other hepatobiliary procedures need validation of numbers for liver resections.

Robotic hepatectomy has a definitive advantage for resection in difficult-to-reach positions such as posterior and superior segments and caudal lobe, sparing the patients of large incisions and speedy postoperative recovery.[12] Augmented reality by image-guided navigational surgery and integrated-infrared fluoroscopy provides an additional advantage.[13-15]

The disadvantage of the robot remains in the huge size of the robotic system and separation of the surgeon and patient.[16] Cost of the instruments and availability of the appropriate size instruments is yet another disadvantage which needs to be taken care of to popularize robotic surgeries in pediatric age group in a developing country like India.[16]

While discussing about the expenses, Liu R et al. in their article[16] have suggested that cost of robotic liver resections is on an average 20% higher than open surgery.[16] Other limitation stated in the same article is lack of tactile feedback leading to frequent suture breakage and retracting a postchemotherapy liver as additional challenges in robotic hepatectomy.[16] Nonarticulating harmonic shears make donor robotic hepatectomy difficult because of loss of EndoWrist function.[16] Yet another disadvantage is the need of presence of an assistant if undocking is needed in emergency.[16]

■ TECHNIQUE FOR ROBOT-ASSISTED LIVER RESECTION

The technique for robot-assisted liver resection is as described here.[17]

Patient Positioning and Trocar Placement

The patient is kept in supine position and camera port of 12 mm size is inserted by open method through umbilicus and pneumoperitoneum created with pressure at 10 mm Hg and flow rate of 4 L/min The trocars for first, second, and third robotic arm are then placed at left of midline, right anterior axillary line, and left anterior axillary line, respectively **(Fig. 1)**.

Three steps are clearly defined.

Step 1: Dissection of the Hepatic Hilum

After retrograde cholecystectomy, the dissection begins at the hepatic pedicle and the right hepatic artery is dissected and divided between ligatures or hem-o-lok clips **(Fig. 2)**. The hepatic pedicle is dissected using a combination

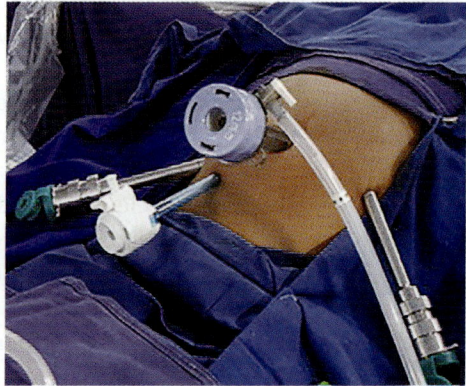

Fig. 1: Port position.

of monopolar hooks and bipolar forceps. The right hepatic artery is dissected first and then cut between hem-o-lok clips **(Figs. 3 and 4)**.

Next, the portal vein is completely dissected with selective stitches and ligatures applied on the posterior branches draining segment 1. The right portal vein is then divided between ligatures or clips.

If the right bile duct is clearly identified extrahepatically, then it is divided approximately 1 cm from the bifurcation. Otherwise, its division is usually done intrahepatically during the resection of the liver parenchyma itself, under indocyanine green (ICG) fluorescence guidance to identify biliary anatomy when in doubt **(Figs. 5 and 6)**

Step 2: Hepatocaval Dissection

The falciform and coronary ligament are divided and lateral reflection of peritoneum dissected along the hepatocaval plane. The inferior surface of liver is retracted to expose the inferior vena cava (IVC).

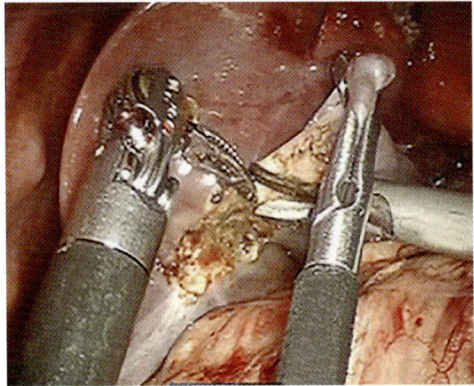

Fig. 2: Dissection begun at the hepatic pedicle.

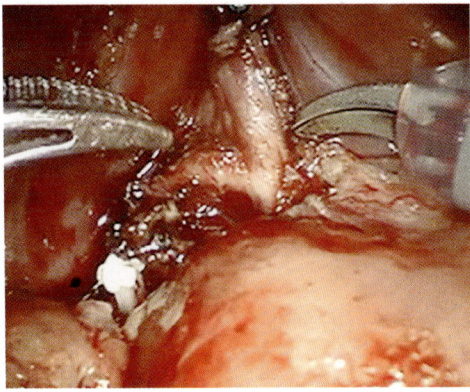

Fig. 3: Division of common hepatic artery into right and left hepatic artery.

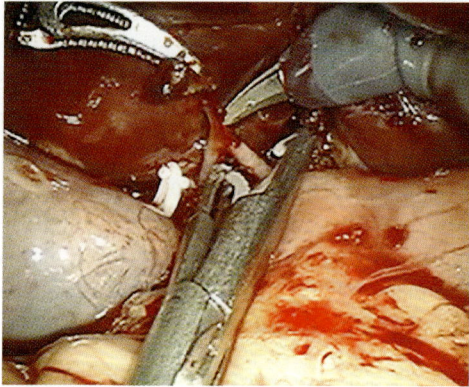

Fig. 4: Right hepatic artery divided between hem-o-lok clips.

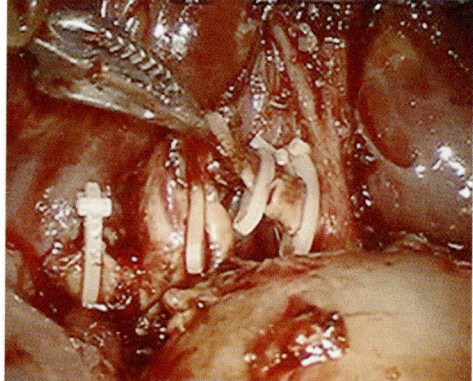

Fig. 5: Division of right hepatic duct.

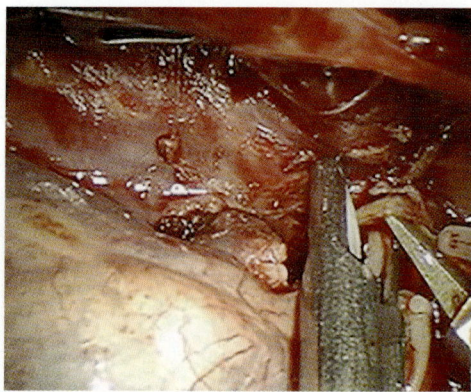

Fig. 6: Division of right portal vein.

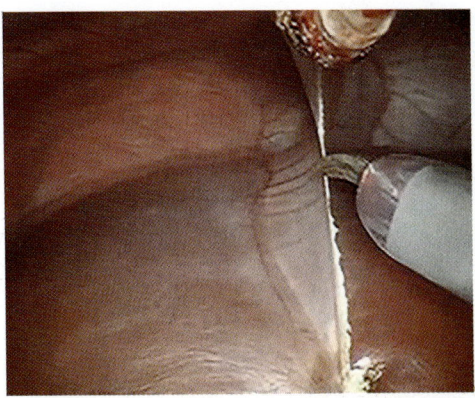

Fig. 7: Dissection continued upto the diaphragm till inferior aspect of right hepatic vein.

The accessory hepatic veins are divided and secured with prolene stitches and/or clips.

The dissection of IVC is continued up to the diaphragm till the inferior aspect of the right hepatic vein is visible. A true "hanging maneuver" may sometimes be needed **(Fig. 7)**.

Step 3: Transection of the Liver

The parenchymal transection of the liver is the last step and follows the ischemic line of demarcation starting at the anterior aspect of liver, along the cholecystocaval line **(Fig. 8)**. The hepatic transection proceeds layer by layer from cortical to subcortical area towards the core using bipolar forceps and robotic harmonic shears as the main tools **(Fig. 9)**. Small bleeders are controlled by electrocautery, while major bleeders require suturing with Prolene stitches and/or hem-o-lok clips. When the dissection reaches to core, then laparoscopic staplers are used to divide the hepatic parenchyma and intracapsular control of the right hepatic vein **(Fig. 10)**. Complete mobilization of liver is then achieved after dividing the remaining peritoneal attachments. The raw hepatic surface is then checked for bleeding and bile leak. Application of fibrin glue is also done by many surgeons over the raw hepatic surface as a sealant. The specimen is retrieved in a specimen bag through a small Pfannenstiel incision and a tube drain is kept in Morrison's pouch **(Fig. 11)**.

The robotic cart is removed from the operative field, pneumoperitoneum is stopped, and the trocars are extracted under direct laparoscopic vision.

■ CONCLUSION

The technical advantages of robot-assisted liver resection are myriad and undeniable.

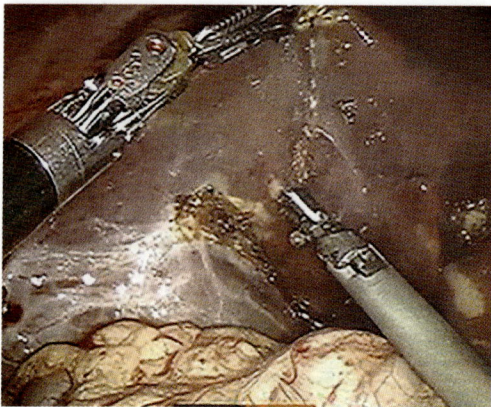

Fig. 8: Demarcation of the liver along the cholecysto-caval line.

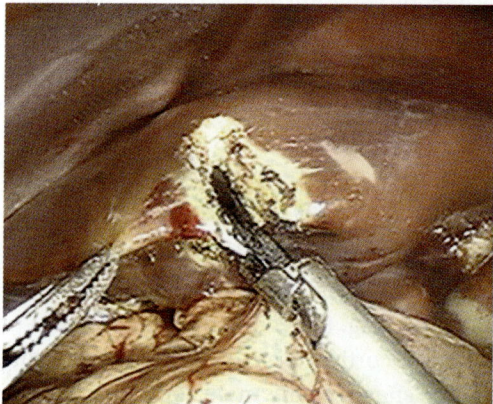

Fig. 9: Hepatic transection in layer by layer fashion using bipolar forceps and harmonic scalpel.

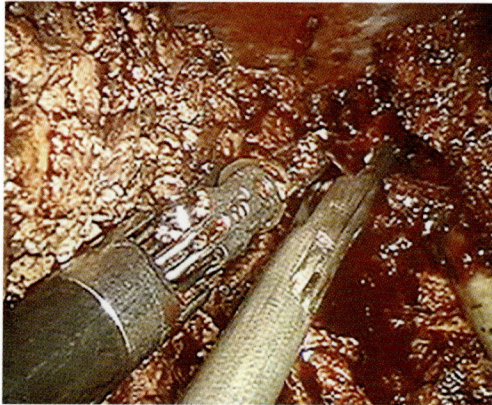

Fig. 10: Intra-capsular control of right hepatic vein.

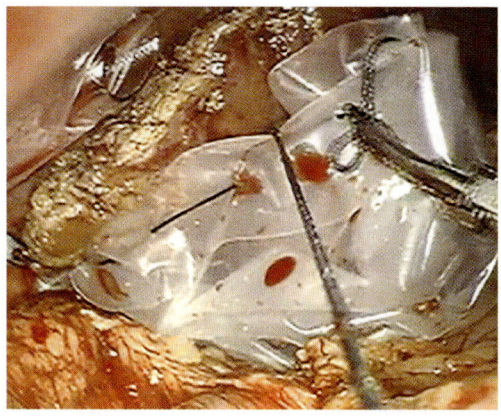

Fig. 11: Specimen extraction in a bag.

In conclusion, with progress in minimal access surgery and advent of robotic surgical systems, the training of hepatobiliary surgeons should also be promoted in robotic surgeries. The robotic system provides safe, quick, and technically easy hepatic resections and also decreases the postoperative morbidities and fastens the recovery time. The availability of small pediatric instruments and cost are the disadvantages which still need to be addressed.

■ REFERENCES

1. Cave J, Clarke S. Paediatric robotic surgery. Ann R Coll Surg Engl. 2018;100 (Suppl 7):18-21.
2. Chen DX, Wang SJ, Jiang YN, Yu MC, Fan JZ, Wang XQ. Robot-assisted gallbladder-preserving hepatectomy for treating S5 hepatoblastoma in a child: A case report and review of the literature. World J Clin Cases. 2019;7(7):872-80.
3. Meehan JJ, Elliott S, Sandler A. The robotic approach to complex hepatobiliary anomalies in children: preliminary report. J Pediatr Surg. 2007;42(12):2110-14.
4. Pham HD, Okata Y, Vu HM, Tran NX, Nguyen QT, Nguyen LT. Robotic-assisted surgery for choledochal cyst in children: early experience at Vietnam National Children's Hospital. Pediatr Surg Int. 2019;35(11):1211-6.
5. Tabrizian P, Midulla PS. Laparoscopic excision of a large hepatic cyst. JSLS. 2010;14:272-4.
6. Dutta S, Nehra D, Woo R, Cohen I. Laparoscopic resection of a benign liver tumor in a child. J Pediatr Surg. 2007;42:1141-5.
7. Oh PS, Hirose S, Parakh S, Cowles RA. Laparoscopic excision of an antenatally diagnosed large simple hepatic cyst in the newborn. Pediatr Surg Int. 2012;28:719-23.
8. Yoon YS, Han HS, Choi YS, Lee SI, Jang JY, Suh KS, et al. Total laparoscopic left lateral sectionectomy performed in a child with benign liver mass. J Pediatr Surg. 2006;41:e25-8.
9. Kim T, Kim DY, Cho MJ, Kim SC, Seo JJ, Kim IK. Surgery for hepatoblastoma: from laparoscopic resection to liver transplantation. Hepatogastroenterology. 2011;58:896-9.

10. Kim T, Kim DY, Cho MJ, Kim SC, Seo JJ, Kim IK. Use of laparoscopic surgical resection for pediatric malignant solid tumors: a case series. Surg Endosc. 2011;25:1484-8.
11. Veenstra MA, Koffron AJ. Minimally-invasive liver resection in pediatric patients: initial experience and outcomes. HPB (Oxford). 2016;18(6):518-22.
12. Guerra F, Di Marino M, Coratti A. Robotic surgery of the liver and biliary tract. J Laparoendosc Adv Surg Tech A. 2019;29(2):141-6.
13. Soler L, Nicolau S, Pessaux P, Mutter D, Marescaux J. Real-time 3D image reconstruction guidance in liver resection surgery Hepatobiliary Surg Nutr. 2014;3(2):73-81.
14. Giulianotti PC, Bianco FM, Daskalaki D, Ciccarelli LFG, Kim J, Benedetti E. Robotic liver surgery: technical aspects and review of the literature. Hepatobiliary Surg Nutr. 2016;5(4):311-21.
15. Rossi G, Tarasconi A, Baiocchi G, Angelis GLD, Gayani F, Mario FD. Fluorescence guided surgery in liver tumors: applications and advantages. Acta Biomed. 2018;89(9-S):135-40.
16. Liu R, Wakabayashi G, Kim HJ, Choi JH, Fong Y, He J, et al. International consensus statement on robotic hepatectomy surgery in 2018. World J Gastroenterol. 2019;25(12):1432-44.
17. Sucandy I, Durrani H, Ross S, Rosemurgy A. Technical approach of robotic total right hepatic lobectomy: How we do it? J Robot Surg. 2019;13(20):193-9.

CHAPTER 12

Minimal Access and Robotic Surgery for Cystic Neoplasms of Pancreatic Body and Tail: Current Perspective

Amir Mushtaq Parray, Ravindra Vats, Deep Goel

■ PROBLEM STATEMENT

Pancreatic cystic neoplasms (PCNs) have changed the face of modern pancreatic surgery. The resections for these tumors have increased from 5 to 15–20% in the last decade. With the significant increase in the use of high-resolution cross-sectional imaging, there has been a considerable increase in the incidental diagnosis of these tumors, particularly in the elderly population posing significant management challenges to the treating physician. Whereas intraductal papillary mucinous neoplasm (IPMN) is precancerous, mucinous cystic neoplasms (MCNs) and solid pseudopapillary neoplasms (SPNs) can progress to cancer; serous cystic neoplasms (SCNs) are mostly benign.[1-7] Management strategies are complex and may range from life-long surveillance to standard oncological or parenchyma-sparing pancreatic resections. Poor preoperative diagnostic accuracy may result in over- or undertreatment.[1,2] This chapter specifically focuses on the current status of minimally invasive surgery in cystic neoplasms localized to the body and tail of the pancreas. The classification and characteristics of the PCNs are summarized in **Table 1** and **Box 1**.

■ CURRENT STATUS OF MINIMALLY INVASIVE PANCREATIC SURGERY

Minimally invasive pancreatic surgery has significantly evolved since its introduction in the 1990s along with other minimally invasive gastrointestinal cancers.[8-13] Some randomized controlled trials and numerous retrospective studies have demonstrated significant advantages of minimally invasive pancreatic resections. Recent international consensus guidelines suggest that minimally invasive pancreatic surgery is at par with open surgery when performed in high-volume centers. However, there are significant concerns regarding increased conversion rates, bleeding, and inferior oncological outcomes at low-volume centers questioning generalized applicability.[8-14] Regarding cystic tumors of the pancreas, the data available is completely skewed as there are no prospective or randomized studies that specifically address these tumors, so the literature available is from either

TABLE 1: Demography, clinical features, and imaging characteristics of pancreatic cystic neoplasms.

	Serous cystic neoplasms (SCNs)	Intraductal papillary mucinous neoplasms (IPMNs)	Mucinous cystic neoplasms (MCNs)	Solid pseudopapillary neoplasms (SPNs)
Demographic characteristics	• Females: 5–7th decade • Incidental or pain in abdomen or mass effect	• No gender predominance: 5–7th decade • Incidental or pain in abdomen or malignancy related	• Females: 5–7th decade • Incidental or pancreatitis or pancreatic insufficiency or malignancy related	• Females: 2–3rd decade • Incidental or abdominal pain or mass effect
Radiological characteristics	• Microcystic honeycomb pattern • Stellate scar • Central calcifications—starburst appearance	• Macrocystic ductal involvement– main duct: Dilated, tortuous main pancreatic duct • Branch duct: Lobulated lesion with grape-like clusters	• Typically unilocular but can be multilocular, macrocystic • Body/tail of the pancreas • No duct communication • Peripheral "eggshell" calcifications	• Partial, cystic mass surrounded by a thick, irregular, contrast-enhancing capsule • In 30% solid tumor areas may be calcified
Pathological characteristics	• Cuboidal cells positive for glycogen; yield <50% • CEA <5–20 ng/mL in majority	• Columnar cells with atypia • Positive for mucin; yield <50% • High yield of malignancy from solid component • CA-19-9 >200 ng/mL in 75% of lesions	• Columnar cells with variable atypia positive for mucin; yield <50% • High yield of malignancy from solid component • CEA >200 ng/mL in approximately 75% of lesions	• Characteristic branching papillae with myxoid stroma • High-yield malignancy from solid component
Genomic characteristics	Allelic loss affecting chromosome 3p and VHL mutation specific	K-ras mutation specific (>90%), not sensitive (<50%) TP53, PTEN, PIK3CA, high DNA amount or high-amplitude allelic loss seen in malignancy	K-ras and GNAS mutation specific (>90%), not sensitive (<50%) TP53, PTEN, PIK3CA, high DNA amount or high-amplitude allelic loss seen in malignancy	CTNNB1 mutation specific

Contd...

Contd...

	Serous cystic neoplasms (SCNs)	Intraductal papillary mucinous neoplasms (IPMNs)	Mucinous cystic neoplasms (MCNs)	Solid pseudopapillary neoplasms (SPNs)
Treatment guidelines	Resect if symptomatic	• Jaundice • Positive cytology (malignancy/HGD) • Solid mass • Growth rate ≥5 mm/year • Increased serum CA 19-9 (>37 U/mL) • Enhancing mural nodule <5 mm	• Jaundice • Pancreatitis • Enhancing mural nodule >5 mm • Pancreatic duct dilation >10 mm • Growth rate >5 mm/2 years • Increased serum level of CA 19-9 • Pancreatic duct dilation 5–9 mm • Cyst diameter >30 mm • Enhancing mural nodule <5 mm • Thickened/enhancing cyst walls • Abrupt change in caliber of pancreatic duct with distal pancreatic atrophy • Lymphadenopathy	Resection

(CA: carbohydrate antigen; CEA: carcinoembryonic antigen; DNA: deoxyribonucleic acid; VHL: Von Hippel–Lindau)

BOX 1: Classification of pancreatic cystic neoplasms.

- *Epithelial (neoplastic)*
  - Intraductal papillary mucinous neoplasm all types
  - Mucinous cystic neoplasm
  - Serous cystic neoplasm
  - Serous cystadenocarcinoma
  - Cystic neuroendocrine tumor grades 1–2
  - Acinar cell cystadenoma
  - Cystic acinar cell carcinoma
  - Solid pseudopapillary neoplasm
  - Cystic ductal adenocarcinoma
  - Cystic pancreatoblastoma
- *Epithelial (non-neoplastic)*
  - Lymphoepithelial cyst
  - Mucinous non-neoplastic cyst
  - Enterogeneous cyst
  - Retention cyst/dysontogenetic cyst
  - Periampullary duodenal wall cyst
  - Endometrial cyst
  - Congenital cyst (in malformation syndromes)

a subgroup analysis of prospective trials or heterogeneous center-specific retrospective studies. European guidelines have recommended a minimally invasive approach as "suitable" for cystic tumors of the pancreas as well as parenchyma-sparing procedures like enucleation in selected cases.[7-38]

Distal pancreatic resections are more commonly adopted as they are less complex and do not require reconstruction when compared to the right-sided resections, i.e., pancreaticoduodenectomy (PD). The evidence for minimally invasive distal pancreatectomy is mainly from single-center studies performed for numerous neoplastic and non-neoplastic etiologies. Comparable outcomes have been demonstrated in terms of operative time, postoperative morbidity and mortality along with less blood loss and shorter hospital stay.[15-32] Even though the LEOPARD-1 trial reported increased operative time for a minimally invasive approach, LAPOP (Comparison of the duration of hospital stay After Laparoscopic or Open distal Pancreatectomy), a randomized controlled trial, along with several meta-analyses reported similar operative times; this is likely due to increased adaptation and negotiation of the learning curve. Both the LEOPARD-1 trial and the LAPOP trial along with a meta-analysis from Nakamura and Nakashima have reported functionally better outcomes with minimally invasive pancreatic resections. These trials along with the Cochrane review have reported equivalent rates of postoperative pancreatic fistula (POPF).[33-36] Studies have reported poorer outcomes following conversion to open surgery, which highlights the importance of preoperative planning and appropriate patient selection. General trends from retrospective and propensity-matching studies have shown equivalent short-term oncological outcomes and long-term outcomes like R0 resections, lymph node yield, and similar rates of median overall survival and 5-year survival rates.[14-36] To put forward the evidence-based guidelines, two international conferences were held in Sao Paulo in Brazil in 2016 and Miami, USA, in 2019, respectively. Miami guidelines have reported equivalent oncological outcomes between open and minimally invasive distal pancreatic resections for pancreatic ductal adenocarcinoma; however, given the scarcity of data available from randomized controlled trials, this recommendation is considered weak.[37,38]

Robotic pancreatic surgery is evolving, although, in a worldwide survey that included 435 surgeons, 79% replied in favor of minimally invasive surgery, and only 9% replied in favor of robotic surgery. Niu et al. in a meta-analysis and Liu et al. in a propensity-matching retrospective study reported a short length of stay in robotic distal pancreatectomy when compared to the laparoscopic approach. Xourafas et al. and Liu et al. have reported significantly lower conversion rates in the robotic approach, particularly in larger sized tumors, signifying the importance of robotic resection in tumors closer to the vessels.[39-42]

Regarding PCNs, there are specific concerns regarding the size of the lesion, histopathology, and the site of the lesion. Ohtsuka et al. in their study documented the safety of minimally invasive resection in patients with MCNs larger than 4.5 cm (up to 13 cm). Margin optimization and cosmetic advantages are other significant factors that may be guaranteed by a minimally invasive approach at high-volume centers.[43] Even though cystic tumors have not been specifically addressed in prospective studies, the analysis of the population-based minimally invasive pancreatic surgery registries shows that cystic tumors constitute >50% of benign tumors.[14,44]

■ PREOPERATIVE DECISION-MAKING

Management decisions in PCNs are complex because of the significant morphological overlap between benign and malignant cysts. However, in addition to the radiological or clinical suspicion of the malignancy, the final decision should be driven by patient factors like age, comorbidity, life expectancy, performance status, and type of surgery offered (pancreatico-duodenectomy vs. distal pancreaticosplenectomy or pancreas-sparing resections). Each surgical decision should be individualized based on the patient and disease factors evaluated in cohesion.[1-4]

Surgery is indicated in patients who are significantly symptomatic due to cysts (cyst-related pancreatitis or obstructive jaundice), cysts with malignant features or cytology suggestive of malignancy, and cysts with malignant potential (MCN, SPN, main-duct IPMN). There has been significant evolution in the treatment of IPMN, whereas branch-duct (BD) IPMN without high-risk stigmata with a size <3 cm may undergo surveillance; if the diagnosis of SCN is established, the decision regarding surgery should be based on associated symptoms, local growth, and progression. Patients who undergo resections for premalignant or potentially malignant cysts like IPMN, SPN, or MCN should undergo margin negative resections with appropriate lymphadenectomy. Parenchyma-sparing surgeries should be limited to selected patients of SCNs, MCNs, or BD IPMN.[3-7]

MINIMALLY INVASIVE APPROACHES IN PANCREATIC CYSTIC NEOPLASMS OF PANCREATIC BODY AND TAIL

Patient Selection

Once the decision to operate has been made, the decision regarding the approach should be individualized, based on the patient and surgeon factors. Whereas most of the high-volume centers would offer a minimally invasive approach to all the patients irrespective of the pathology in the absence of surrounding organ invasion, center-specific and surgeon-specific modifications of the indications may be based on the body mass index (BMI) of the patients, comorbidity status, previous abdominal operations, or history of severe pancreatitis. Theoretically, a minimally invasive approach may be offered to all the patients with cystic tumors in the pancreatic body and tail. Small deeper tumors are preoperative marked with ink during preoperative endoscopic ultrasonography (treatment algorithm; **Flowchart 1**).[14,44-46]

Flowchart 1: Management algorithm for pancreatic cystic neoplasms.

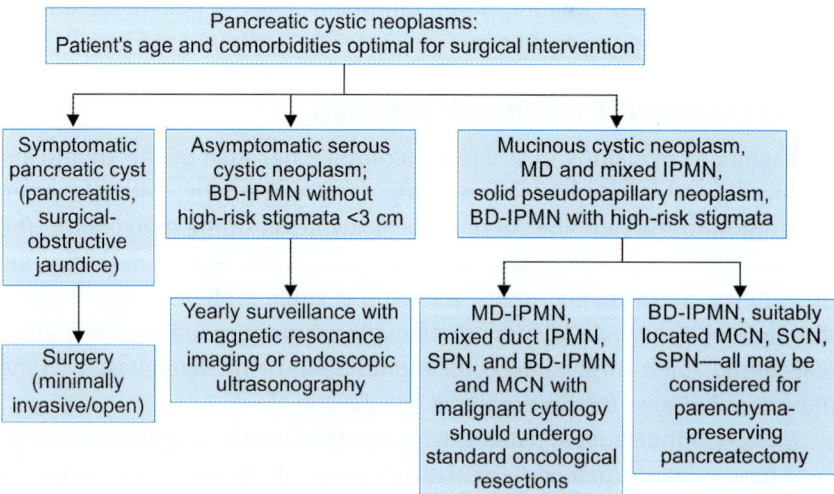

(BD-IPMN: branch duct intraductal papillary mucinous neoplasia; MCN: mucinous cystic neoplasm; MD-IPMN: main duct-IPMN; SCN: serous cystic neoplasm; SPN: solid pseudopapillary neoplasm)

General Principles

The safety and efficacy of minimally invasive distal pancreatic resections have been established in numerous center-specific studies and selected randomized controlled trials. With a median conversion rate of 12% (0–32%) across the studies, bleeding, proximity to major vessels, male sex, increased visceral fat, and failure to progress are considered the predictors of conversion to open surgery. Conversion, if required, should be done early to maintain the oncological efficacy of the procedure and decrease the complications attributed to delayed conversion. Splenic preservation should be considered in selected cases of PCNs given the limited lymphadenectomy required; however, the final decision should be made based on the intraoperative ease.[14,44-48] Various studies by Kang et al. and Worhunsky et al. have reported the safety of laparoscopic spleen preserving distal pancreatectomy. Apart from increased operative duration, increased pancreatic resection volumes, and transient splenic ischemia in Warshaw's techniques, studies have reported equivalent outcomes when compared to the vessel preservation technique.[49,50] Giulianotti et al. in their study reported increased safety and success in the preservation of the spleen during distal pancreatic resections using a robotic platform.[51]

Many surgeons have proposed the use of a 5–7 cm epigastric hand-port to decrease the learning curve associated with this procedure and increase the ease associated with the procedure. Similarly, approaching the medial part of the pancreas and establishing early control of splenic vessels at the medial aspect via a lesser sac approach is preferred by some surgeons.[52-55] Yao et al. and Huagvik et al. in their studies of single-incision laparoscopic distal pancreatectomy reported equivalent outcomes when compared to the multiport approach.[56,57]

Parenchyma-sparing Procedures

The clinical impact of the PCNs is related to their malignant potential. SCNs do not have any malignant potential, so they are rarely mentioned in the surgical literature. They constitute 20% of all PCNs and tend to occur predominantly in elderly females. Since treatment is related to the symptoms, size, and progression of the lesion, suitably located lesions may be subjected to parenchyma-sparing procedures like segmental pancreatectomy or spleen preserving distal pancreatectomy. MCNs are considered premalignant and transformation occurs in 50% of patients via adenoma–carcinoma sequence. These patients should preferably undergo formal pancreatic resections; however, based on the location and if intraoperative frozen section establishes no malignancy, parenchyma-sparing procedures may be offered.[58-67] Main duct and mixed-type IPMNs are associated with malignant transformation in 70% of patients; as such, they warrant formal oncological resections. BD IPMNs have limited but relevant malignant potential and prevention of the malignancy is the priority in these cases; after proper assessment of imaging and cytological features, they may be considered for enucleation and other parenchyma-sparing procedures based on tumor location and size. SPNs may be offered standard pancreatic resections or central pancreatectomy depending on the location of the tumor.[68-74]

Enucleation

All the patients who are planned for enucleation should be adequately counseled about the prospective change to standard resection based on the intraoperative findings. Although clinical evidence is limited, surgical enucleation should be considered in patients with tumor size not >2 cm and a distance of >3 mm from the main duct. A preoperative magnetic resonance cholangiopancreatography and intraoperative ultrasonography are essential investigations required. For slightly deeper located tumors, preoperative main pancreatic duct stenting may be considered. In BD IPMN, it is important to identify the communicating duct and send it for an intraoperative frozen section to rule out invasive carcinoma and high-grade dysplasia, and subsequently, securely ligate the duct. Although the literature is limited, minimally invasive approaches have been safely adopted in pancreatic enucleation. Pancreatic enucleation may be associated with an increased risk of POPF (up to 43–45%) and predictive factors associated with increased POPF include high BMI, cyst morphology, cyst to duct distance of <3 mm, and previous history of acute pancreatitis.[58-63]

Central Pancreatectomy

Central pancreatectomy is indicated in patients with tumors located in the pancreatic neck and body without any surrounding organ invasion or gastroduodenal artery involvement, typically in patients where >5 cm of the distal pancreas can be preserved. Although central pancreatectomy is predominantly offered mainly for patients with neuroendocrine tumors, recently it is increasingly being offered to patients with BD IPMN, mucinous cystadenomas, and solid pseudopapillary tumors. Preoperative cross-sectional imaging is essential to establish the relationship of the tumor with the gastroduodenal artery. Intraoperatively, every effort should be made to preserve the gastroduodenal artery and the need for sacrificing should be considered as an indication for conversion into standard pancreaticoduodenectomy. The left-sided pancreatic remnant should be drained as pancreaticojejunostomy or pancreaticogastrostomy. There is significant data to suggest that central pancreatectomy allows for better preservation of pancreatic function, but associated complications are relatively higher. To optimize the outcomes, central pancreatectomy should be selectively offered to the young nondiabetic patients, with a distal pancreatic remnant of >5 cm and computed tomography (CT) features suggestive of a low-risk pancreas. The incidence of POPF post central pancreatectomy may range from 20 to 70%.[64-67]

Functional Outcomes

Parenchyma-preserving pancreatic resections offer excellent long-term exocrine and endocrine functional outcomes. Standard pancreatic resections are associated with a 10–20% incidence of new-onset endocrine dysfunction and more than 20% of patients will need pancreatic enzyme supplementations. Pancreatic parenchymal-preserving resections are rarely associated with new-onset exocrine or endocrine dysfunction. Both enucleation and central pancreatectomy provide excellent quality of life.[48,71-73]

■ TECHNICAL ASPECTS

Patients may be variably placed in supine, lithotomy, or lateral position depending on the center and surgeon preferences. The majority of the surgery is performed in slight Trendelenburg's position with the left side rotated upward. Surgery is performed using four to six upper abdominal ports, with the umbilicus as the camera port and the rest of the ports along the mid-axillary and mid-clavicular lines. The left lobe of the liver is retracted using Nathanson's retractor or suture retraction. In Xi Da Vinci Robotic platform, four ports are placed in a straight line at the level of the umbilicus. One or two assistant ports may be placed based on surgeon's preferences **(Figs. 1 and 2)**.

Operative Technique for Distal Pancreatectomy

The spleen-preservation technique is adopted whenever feasible. Gastrolysis is done close to the stomach to avoid overhanging omentum during dissection. The stomach is either retracted or suture fixed to the anterior abdomen wall. Pancreatic dissection is started along the inferior border of the pancreas. This is followed by splenic flexure mobilization. If splenectomy is planned, it is preferable to mobilize the distal pancreaticosplenic region at this time of the operation. This is more important while doing robotic surgery as this step may become exceedingly difficult in the latter part of the surgery. This is followed by dorsal dissection along the splenic artery. A tunnel is created above the splenic vein depending on the location of the tumor. A suitable stapler is used to divide the pancreas. While applying the stapler, an appropriate staple height should be chosen based on the pancreatic thickness and sequential gradual compression should be followed before firing the stapler. The rest of the dissection is completed and the specimen

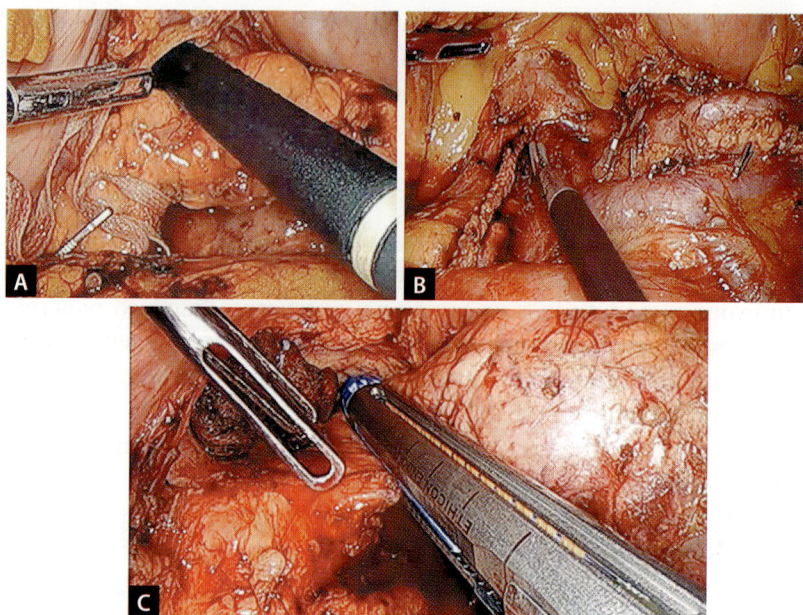

Figs. 1A to C: Laparoscopic distal pancreatectomy. (A) Use of laparoscopic intraoperative ultrasonography; (B) Vessel preservation in Spleen preserving distal pancreatectomy; (C) Proximal stapled division in large cystic tumor of body and tail of the pancreas.

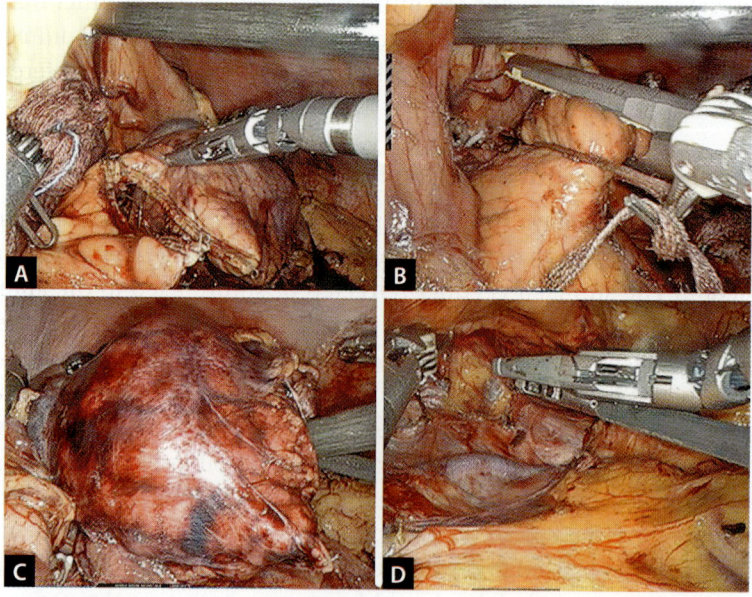

Figs. 2A to D: Robotic distal pancreatectomy. (A and B) Proximal pancreatic division using a stapler; (C) Mobilized distal tumor; (D) Posterior dissection ensuring clear posterior margins.

is removed in a specimen bag via Pfennelstein or natural orifice based on the surgeon's experience. A closed suction drain should be placed at the cut surface of the pancreas. In cases where the spleen is preserved, care should be taken regarding the bleeding along the splenic vessels if they are preserved and the vascularity of the spleen in the case where Warshaw's technique was used.[17-37]

Operative Technique for Parenchyma-sparing Procedures

Appropriate localization is necessary before enucleation along with intraoperative laparoscopic ultrasonography. Three to four ports are placed in the same configuration as above. After gastrolysis, the site is identified from previously injected ink. Intraoperatively location and relation to the main pancreatic duct are documented using intraoperative ultrasonography. Enucleation is done using ultrasonic dissection or by using monopolar or bipolar dissecting devices. The residual cavity should be drained to avoid postoperative collections. Some surgeons use sealants to pack the residual cavity.[58-63]

Segmental pancreatic resections like central pancreatectomy involve two transection surfaces: one at the level of superior mesenteric vein/portal vein (SMV)/PV level and the other distally. Care should be exercised to preserve the gastroduodenal artery. Reconstruction is completed using various techniques like proximal end closure and distal pancreaticojejunostomy or double anastomosis or pancreaticogastrostomy. Drainage should be established given the relatively higher risk of POPF.[64-67]

■ PROGNOSIS AND FOLLOW-UP

The prognosis is excellent. In SCNs, follow-up surveillance is rarely indicated as recurrence is extremely rare. Mucinous neoplasms including IPMNs have excellent survival rates ranging up to 95% 10-year survival rates. All mucinous tumors require lifelong follow-up of the pancreatic remnant by either annual MRI or endoultrasonography. Repeated resections are required in IPMN recurrences to improve survival and avoid malignancy.[74-78]

■ CONCLUSION

Minimally invasive distal pancreatic resection is being increasingly used for cystic tumors of the pancreas with comparable results to open surgery. Given the excellent prognosis and advanced technical demands associated with pancreatic surgery and at the same time trend toward parenchyma-sparing procedures, minimally invasive approaches need to be selectively evaluated for cystic pancreatic tumors in terms of long-term outcomes. In high-volume centers and in experienced hands, these procedures may provide excellent short-term and long-term outcomes. Further data from randomized controlled trials would provide definitive answers.

■ REFERENCES

1. Tanaka M, Castillo CF, Adsay V, Chari S, Falconi M, Jang JY, et al. International consensus guidelines 2012 for the management of IPMN and MCN of the pancreas. Pancreatology. 2012;12:183-97.
2. Tanaka M, Castillo CF, Kamisawa T, Jang JY, Levy P, Otsuka T, et al. Revisions of international consensus Fukuoka guidelines for the management of IPMN of the pancreas. Pancreatology. 2017;17:738-53.
3. European Study Group on Cystic Tumours of the Pancreas. European evidence-based guidelines on pancreatic cystic neoplasms. Gut. 2018;67(5):789-804.
4. Elta GH, Enestvedt BK, Sauer BG, Lennon AM. ACG clinical guideline: diagnosis and management of pancreatic cysts. Am J Gastroenterol. 2018;113:464-79.
5. Megibow AJ, Baker ME, Morgan DE, Kamel IR, Sahani DV, Newman E, et al. Management of incidental pancreatic cysts: a white paper of the ACR incidental findings committee. J Am Coll Radiol. 2017;14:911-23.
6. van Huijgevoort NCM, Chiaro MD, Wolfgang CL, Hooft JE, Besselink MG. Diagnosis and management of pancreatic cystic neoplasms: current evidence and guidelines. Nat Rev Gastroenterol Hepatol. 2019;16(11):676-89.
7. Jais B, Rebours V, Malleo G, Salvia R, Montana M, Maggino L, et al. Serous cystic neoplasm of the pancreas: a multinational study of 2622 patients under the auspices of the International Association of Pancreatology and European Pancreatic Club (European Study Group on Cystic Tumors of the Pancreas). Gut. 2016;65(2):305-12.
8. Kim HH, Han SU, Kim MC, Kim W, Lee HJ, Ryu SW, et al. Effect of laparoscopic distal gastrectomy vs open distal gastrectomy on long-term survival among patients with stage i gastric cancer: The KLASS-01 randomized clinical trial. JAMA Oncol. 2019;5(4):506-13.
9. van der Pas MH, Haglind E, Cuesta MA, Lacy AM, Hop WC, Bonjer HJ, et al. Laparoscopic versus open surgery for rectal cancer (COLOR II): short-term outcomes of a randomised, phase 3 trial. Lancet Oncol. 2013;14(3):210-8.
10. Park JW, Kang SB, Hao J, Lim SB, Choi HS, Kim DW, et al. Open versus laparoscopic surgery for mid or low rectal cancer after neoadjuvant chemoradiotherapy (COREAN trial): 10-year follow-up of an open-label, non-inferiority, randomised controlled trial. Lancet Gastroenterol Hepatol. 2021;6(7):569-77.
11. Gagner M, Pomp A. Laparoscopic pylorus-preserving pancreatoduodenectomy. Surg Endosc. 1994;8(5):408-10.
12. Cuschieri A. Laparoscopic pancreatic resections. semin laparosc surg. 1996; 3:15-20.
13. Joseph B, Morton JM, Hernandez-Boussard T, Rubinfeld I, Faraj C, Valenovivh V. Relationship between hospital volume, system clinical resources, and mortality in pancreatic resection. J Am Coll Surg. 2009;208(4):520-7.
14. Siech M, Bartsch D, Beger HG, Benz S, Bergman U, Busch P, et al. Indications for laparoscopic pancreas operations: results of a consensus conference and the previous laparoscopic pancreas register. Surgeon. 2012;83(3):247-53.
15. Bhandare MS, Parray A, Chaudhari VA, Shrikhande SV. Minimally invasive surgery for pancreatic cancer-are we there yet? A narrative review. Chin Clin Oncol. 2022;11(1):3.
16. van Hilst J, de Graaf N, Abu Hilal M, Besselink MG. the landmark series: minimally invasive pancreatic resection. Ann Surg Oncol. 2021;28(3):1447-56.

17. Kooby DA, Hawkins WG, Schmidt CM, Weber SM, Bentrem DJ, Gillespie TW, et al. A multicenter analysis of distal pancreatectomy for adenocarcinoma: is laparoscopic resection appropriate? J Am Coll Surg. 2010;210(5):779-85,786-7.
18. Magge D, Gooding W, Choudry H, Steve J, Steel J, Hughes SJ, et al. Comparative effectiveness of minimally invasive and open distal pancreatectomy for ductal adenocarcinoma. JAMA Surg. 2013;148:525-31.
19. Hu M, Zhao G, Wang F, Zhao Z, Li C, Liu R. Laparoscopic versus open distal splenopancreatectomy for the treatment of pancreatic body and tail cancer: a retrospective, mid-term follow-up study at a single academic tertiary care institution. Surg Endosc. 2014;28:2584-91.
20. Rehman S, John SK, Lochan R, Jacques BC, Manas DM, Charnley RM, et al. Oncological feasibility of laparoscopic distal pancreatectomy for adenocarcinoma: a single-institution comparative study. World J Surg. 2014; 38(2):476-83.
21. Lee SH, Kang CM, Hwang HK, Choi SH, Lee WJ, Chi HS. Minimally invasive RAMPS in well-selected left-sided pancreatic cancer within Yonsei criteria: long-term (>median 3 years) oncologic outcomes. Surg Endosc. 2014;28:2848-55.
22. Shin SH, Kim SC, Song KB, Hwang DW, Lee JH, Lee D, et al. A comparative study of laparoscopic vs. open distal pancreatectomy for left-sided ductal adenocarcinoma: a propensity score matched analysis. J Am Coll Surg. 2015;220(2):177-85.
23. Sulpice L, Farges O, Goutte N, Bendersky N, Dokmak S, Sauvanet A, et al. laparoscopic distal pancreatectomy for pancreatic ductal adenocarcinoma: time for a randomized controlled trial? results of an all-inclusive national observational study. Ann Surg. 2015;262(5):868-73; discussion 873-4.
24. Sharpe SM, Talamonti MS, Wang E, Bentrem DJ, Roggin KK, Prinz RA, et al. The laparoscopic approach to distal pancreatectomy for ductal adenocarcinoma results in shorter lengths of stay without compromising oncologic outcomes. Am J Surg. 2015;209(3):557-63.
25. Zhang M, Fang R, Mou Y, Chen R, Xu X, Zhang R, et al. LDP vs ODP for pancreatic adenocarcinoma: a case-matched study from a single-institution. BMC Gastroenterol 2015;15:182.
26. Stauffer JA, Coppola A, Mody K, Asbun HJ. Laparoscopic versus open distal pancreatectomy for pancreatic adenocarcinoma. World J Surg. 2016;40:1477-84.
27. Anderson KL Jr, Adam MA, Thomas S, Roman SA, Sosa JA. Impact of minimally invasive vs. open distal pancreatectomy on use of adjuvant chemoradiation for pancreatic adenocarcinoma. Am J Surg. 2017;213(4):601-5.
28. Plotkin A, Ceppa EP, Zarzaur BL, Kilbane EM, Riall TS, Pitt HA. Reduced morbidity with minimally invasive distal pancreatectomy for pancreatic adenocarcinoma. HPB (Oxford). 2017;19:279-85.
29. Kantor O, Bryan DS, Talamonti MS, Lutfi W, Sharpe S, Winchester DJ, et al. laparoscopic distal pancreatectomy for cancer provides oncologic outcomes and overall survival identical to open distal pancreatectomy. J Gastrointest Surg. 2017;21:1620-5.
30. Bauman MD, Becerra DG, Kilbane EM, Zyromski MJ, Schmidt TM, Pitt HA, et al. Laparoscopic distal pancreatectomy for pancreatic cancer is safe and effective. Surg Endosc. 2018;32:53-61.
31. Raoof M, Ituarte PHG, Woo Y, Warner SG, Singh G, Fong Y, et al. Propensity score-matched comparison of oncological outcomes between laparoscopic and open distal pancreatic resection. Br J Surg. 2018;105(5):578-86.

32. van Hilst J, de Rooij T, Klompmaker S, Rawashdeh M, Aleotti M, Alseidi A, et al. Minimally invasive versus open distal pancreatectomy for ductal adenocarcinoma (DIPLOMA): A Pan-European propensity score matched study. Ann Surg. 2019;269:10-7.
33. de Rooij T, van Hilst J, van Santvoort H, Boerma D, Daams F, Dejong C, et al. minimally invasive versus open distal pancreatectomy (LEOPARD): A multicenter patient-blinded randomized controlled trial. Ann Surg. 2019; 269(1):2-9.
34. Björnsson B, Larsson AL, Hjalmarsson C, Gasslander T, Sandstrom P. Comparison of the duration of hospital stay after laparoscopic or open distal pancreatectomy: randomized controlled trial. Br J Surg. 2020;107:1281-8.
35. Riviere D, Gurusamy KS, Kooby DA, Vollmer CM, Davidson BR, Besselink MGH, et al. Laparoscopic versus open distal pancreatectomy for pancreatic cancer. Cochrane Database Syst Rev. 2016;4(4):CD011391.
36. Nakamura M, Nakashima H. Laparoscopic distal pancreatectomy and pancreatoduodenectomy: is it worthwhile? A meta-analysis of laparoscopic pancreatectomy. J Hepatobiliary Pancreat Sci. 2013; 20(4):421-28.
37. Vollmer CM, Asbun HJ, Barkun J, Besselink MG, Boggi U, Conlon KCP, et al. Proceedings of the first international state of the art conference on minimally invasive pancreatic resection (MIPR). HPB (Oxford). 2017;19(3):171-77.
38. Asbun HJ, Moekotte AL, Vissers FL, Kunzler F, Cipriani F, Balduzzi A, et al. The Miami International evidence-based guidelines on minimally invasive pancreas resection. Ann Surg. 2020;271(1):1-14.
39. Niu X, Yu B, Yao L, Tian J, Guo T, Ma S, et al. Comparison of surgical outcomes of robot-assisted laparoscopic distal pancreatectomy versus laparoscopic and open resections: a systematic review and meta-analysis. Asian J Surg. 2019; 42(1):32-45.
40. Caba Molina D, Lambreton F, Arrangoiz Majul R. Trends in robotic pancreaticoduodenectomy and distal pancreatectomy. J Laparoendosc Adv Surg Tech. 2019;29(2):147-51.
41. Liu R, Liu Q, Zhao ZM, Tan XL, Gao YX, Zhao GD. Robotic versus laparoscopic distal pancreatectomy: a propensity score-matched study. J Surg Oncol. 2017; 116(4):461-9.
42. Xourafas D, Ashley SW, Clancy TE. Comparison of perioperative outcomes between open, laparoscopic, and robotic distal pancreatectomy: an analysis of 1815 patients from the ACS-NSQIP procedure-targeted pancreatectomy database. J Gastrointest Surg. 2017;21(9):1442-52.
43. Ohtsuka T, Takahata S, Takanami H, Ueda J, Mizumoto K, Shimizu S, et al. Laparoscopic surgery is applicable for larger mucinous cystic neoplasms of the pancreas. J Hepatobiliary Pancreat Sci. 2014;21:343-48.
44. Bosscha K, van Dam RM, van Dieren S, Dijkgraaf MG, van Eijck CH, Gerhards MF, et al. A nationwide comparison of laparoscopic and open distal pancreatectomy for benign and malignant disease. J Am Coll Surg. 2015;220(3):263-70.e1.
45. Chalikonda S, Aguilar-Saavedra JR, Walsh RM. Laparoscopic robotic-assisted pancreaticoduodenectomy: a case-matched comparison with open resection. Surg Endosc. 2012;26:2397-402.
46. Song KB, Kim SC, Park JB, Kim YH, Jung YS, Kim MH, et al. Sing-center experience of laparoscopic left pancreatic resection in 359 consecutive patients:

changing the surgical paradigm of left pancreatic resection. Surg Endosc. 2011;25:3364-72.
47. SH, Lee WJ. Splenic vein thrombosis and pancreatic fistula after minimally invasive distal pancreatectomy. BJS. 2014;101:114-9.
48. Norton JA, Visser BC. Laparoscopic spleen preserving distal pancreatectomy: the technique must suit the lesion. J Gastrointest Surg. 2014;18:1445-51.
49. Kang CM, Chung YE, Jung MJ, Hwang HK, Choi SH, Lee WJ. Splenic vein thrombosis and pancreatic fistula after minimally invasive distal pancreatectomy. Br J Surg. 2014;101:114-9.
50. Worhunsky DJ, Zak Y, Dua MM, Poultsides GA, Norton JA, Visser BC. Laparoscopic spleen preserving distal pancreatectomy: the technique must suit the lesion. J Gastrointest Surg. 2014;18:1445-51.
51. Giulianotti PC, Sbrana F, Bianco FM, Shah G, Addedo P, Coratti A, et al. Robot-assisted laparoscopic pancreatic surgery: single-surgeon experience. Surg Endosc. 2010;24:1646-57.
52. Coit D, Jaques D, Angelica MD, DeGregoris G, Fong Y, Brennan M. Initial experience with hand-assisted laparoscopic distal pancreatectomy. Surg Endosc. 2006;20:142-8.
53. Abe N, Mori T, Sugiyama M. Tips on laparoscopic distal pancreatectomy. J Hepatobiliary Pancreat Sci. 2014;21:e41-7.
54. Sartori CA, Baiocchi GL. Transecting the pancreas neck with electrothermal bipolar vessel sealer (Ligasure) in laparoscopic left pancreatectomy. Surg Laparosc Endosc Percutan Tech. 2009;19:e175-6.
55. Suzuki O, Nakamura F, Ambo Y, Nakamura T, Kishida A, Kashimura N. Lesser curvature approach in laparoscopic distal pancreatectomy. Surg Laparosc Endosc Percutan Tech. 2013;232:e57-60.
56. Yao D, Wu S, Li Y, Chen Y, Yu X, Han J. Transumbilical single-incision laparoscopic distal pancreatectomy: preliminary experience and comparison to conventional multi-port laparoscopic surgery. BMC Surg. 2014;14:105.
57. Haugvik SP, Rosok BI, Waage A, Mathisen O, Edwin B. Single-incision versus conventional laparoscopic distal pancreatectomy: a single-institution case-control study. Langenbecks Arch Surg. 2013;398:1091-6.
58. Lennon AM, Newman N, Makary MA, Edil BH, Shin EJ, Khashab MA, et al. EUS-guided tattooing before laparoscopic distal pancreatic resection (with video). Gastrointest Endosc. 2010;72:1089-94.
59. Pederzoli P. Enucleation of pancreatic neoplasms. Br J Surg. 2007;94:1254-9.
60. Hackert T, Hinz U, Fritz S, Strobel O, Schneider L, Hartwig W, et al. Enucleation in pancreatic surgery: indications, technique, and outcome compared to standard pancreatic resections. Langenbecks Arch Surg. 2011;396:1197–203.
61. Del Chiaro M, Albiin N, Segersvärd R. Enucleation of branch duct-IPMN in a transplant patient. Pancreatology. 2013;13(3):312-3.
62. Turrini O, Schmidt CM, Pitt HA, Guiramand J, Aguilar-Saavedra JR, Aboudi S, et al. Side-branch intraductal papillary mucinous neoplasms of the pancreatic head/ uncinate: resection or enucleation? HPB (Oxford). 2011;13:126-31.
63. Shin LK, Brant-Zawadzki G, Kamaya A, Jeffrey RB. Intraoperative ultrasound of the pancreas. Ultrasound Q. 2009;25(1):39-48.
64. Goudard Y, Gaujoux S, Dokmak S, Cros J, Couvelard A, Palazzo M, Ronot M, et al. Reappraisal of central pancreatectomy a 12-year single-center experience. JAMA Surg. 2014;149:356-63.

65. Müller MW, Friess H, Kleeff J, Hinz U, Wente MN, Paramythiotis D, et al. Middle segmental pancreatic resection: an option to treat benign pancreatic body lesions. Ann Surg. 2006;244:909-18.
66. Kang CM, Lee JH, Lee WJ. Minimally invasive central pancreatectomy: current status and future directions. J Hepatobiliary Pancreat Sci. 2014;21(12):831-40.
67. Song KB, Kim SC, Park KM, Hwang DW, Lee JH, Lee DJ, et al. Laparoscopic central pancreatectomy for benign or low-grade malignant lesions in the pancreatic neck and proximal body. Surg Endosc. 2015;29:937-46.
68. Balzano G, Carvello M, Piemonti L, Nano R, Ariotti R, Mercalli A, et al. Combined laparoscopic spleen preserving distal pancreatectomy and islet autotransplantation for benign pancreatic neoplasm. World J Gastroenterol. 2014;20:4030-6.
69. Fatima Z, Ichikawa T, Motosugi U, Muhi A, Sano K, Sou H, et al. Magnetic resonance diffusion-weighted imaging in the characterization of pancreatic mucinous cystic lesions. Clin Radiol. 2011;66(2):108-11.
70. Al-Kurd A, Chapchay K, Grozinsky-Glasberg S, Mazeh H. Laparoscopic resection of pancreatic neuroendocrine tumors. World J Gastroenterol. 2014;20(17):4908-16.
71. Langer P, Fendrich V, Bartsch DK. Minimally invasive resection of neuro-endocrine pancreatic tumors. Chirurg. 2009;80(2):105-12.
72. Gupta V, Bhandare MS, Chaudhari V, Parray A, Shrikhande SV. Organ preserving pancreatic resections offer better long-term conservation of pancreatic function at the expense of high perioperative major morbidity: a fair trade-off for benign or low malignant potential pancreatic neoplasms-a single-center experience. Langenbecks Arch Surg. 2022;407(4):1507-15.
73. DiNorcia J, Lee MK, Reavey PL, Genkinger JM, Lee JA, Schrope BA, et al. One hundred and thirty resections for pancreatic neuroendocrine tumor: evaluating the impact of minimally invasive and parenchyma-sparing techniques. J Gastrointest Surg. 2010;14:1536-46.
74. Larghi A, Panic N, Capurso G, Leoncini E, Arzani D, Salvia R, et al. Prevalence and risk factors of extrapancreatic malignancies in a large cohort of patients with intraductal papillary mucinous neoplasm (IPMN) of the pancreas. Ann Oncol. 2013;24(7):1907-11.
75. Reid-Lombardo KM, Mathis KL, Wood CM, Harmsen WS, Sarr MG. Frequency of extrapancreatic neoplasms in intraductal papillary mucinous neoplasm of the pancreas: implications for management. Ann Surg. 2010;251:64-9.
76. Wasif N, Bentrem DJ, Farrell JJ, Ko CY, Hines OJ, Reber HA, et al. Invasive intraductal papillary mucinous neoplasm versus sporadic pancreatic adenocarcinoma: a stage-matched comparison of outcomes. Cancer. 2010;116:3369-77.
77. Poultsides GA, Reddy S, Cameron JL, Hruban RH, Pawlik TM, Ahuja N, et al. Histopathologic basis for the favorable survival after resection of intra-ductal papillary mucinous neoplasm associated invasive adenocarcinoma of the pancreas. Ann Surg. 2010;251:470-6.
78. Turrini O, Waters JA, Schnelldorfer T, Lillemoe KD, Yiannoutsos CT, Farnell MB, et al. Invasive intraductal papillary mucinous neoplasm: predictors of survival and role of adjuvant therapy. HPB (Oxford). 2010;12:447-55.

CHAPTER 13

Robotic-assisted Revision Bariatric Surgery

Arun Kumar, Vitish Singla, Prasanna Ramana, Sandeep Aggarwal

■ INTRODUCTION

Over the last two decades, bariatric surgery has established itself as the favorable option of sustainable weight loss measure among the several modalities including lifestyle modifications and pharmacotherapy. With increased safety and efficacy of bariatric procedures over the last decade, the number of patients undergoing primary bariatric procedures has seen a significant rise. However, with long-term results now available, reports of insufficient weight loss, weight regain, or recidivism and that of chronic malnutrition has brought into play the role of revision or conversion bariatric surgery. Unsurprisingly, the need for reoperative bariatric procedures has also increased progressively over the years. As per one report, revision surgery comprises 1 in every 7 of all bariatric procedures in US and may soon exceed the primary gastric bypass procedures.[1] The incidence of reoperative surgery may vary over a wide range of 5–54% depending upon the type of primary procedure with reoperation rates as high as 60% reported with adjustable gastric banding (AGB) and vertical banded gastroplasty (VBG) in the literature.[2-4] Roux-en-Y gastric bypass (RYGB) has a reoperation rate of 2.1–20% while for sleeve gastrectomy (SG), it ranges between 3.3% and 34%.[5,6] Lowest rates of reoperation (5%) had been reported with purely malabsorptive procedures like biliopancreatic diversion (BPD) and BPD with duodenal switch (BPD-DS).[7] Besides the higher rates of primary bariatric surgeries, the increasing trends of reoperative bariatric surgery might be due to inability of some procedures to achieve sustained weight loss, lack of standardization of techniques of different bariatric procedures, a shift in the types of procedures being performed, an increased experience with reoperative cases, and availability of the literature supporting the benefits of reoperation surgery.

Broadly, the reoperations in bariatric surgery are usually indicated in the wake of insufficient weight loss, significant weight regain, persistence or recurrence of obesity-related comorbidities, and complications related to the index procedure, which can be early or late. *Reoperations can be categorized as conversions, revisions or corrective, and reversal:*

- *Conversion:* Change to a different type of procedure from the index procedure, e.g., SG to RYGB or one-anastomosis gastric bypass (OAGB).

- *Revision or corrective:* Modification addressing complications or ineffective treatment of a previous bariatric procedure, e.g., RYGB to distal RYGB, SG to re-SG.
- *Reversal:* Procedures that reestablish the original anatomy, e.g., reversal of OAGB or RYGB.

Reoperative procedures are technically challenging owing to underlying adhesions, inflammation, tissue scarring, and distorted anatomy, at times. This requires a great deal of skill, expertise, and dexterity on the part of operating team, besides the laborious efforts to perform such extensive procedures. Currently, the minimal access approach using the conventional laparoscopy is preferred for primary bariatric surgery due to its obvious advantages of less postoperative pain, shorter hospital stay, and quick recovery. However, when it comes to reoperation, the mandate is divided, as some authors claim the technical advantage of a robot in these arduous procedures despite a higher operative time.[8]

The first robot-assisted RYGB was performed in 2001, a year after the da Vinci robotic surgical system (Intuitive Surgical, Inc., Sunnyvale, California) got the United States Food and Drug Administration (FDA) approval.[9] Soon after, the robotic system was used for advanced procedures expecting enhancements such as instruments with a wrist-like action (seven degrees of freedom), improved ergonomics and three-dimensional vision to increase the patient's safety and reduce the learning curve for surgeons. Since then, almost all the standard bariatric procedures including the gastric banding, RYGB, SG, and the revisional surgeries have been performed robotically with published results revealing diverse experiences and outcomes. Recent studies have demonstrated benefits of routine use of robotic approach, especially in the revisional bariatric surgery (RBS).[10] The aim of this chapter is to discuss the reoperative bariatric surgery and the key aspects of robot-assisted RBS (RRBS), besides reviewing their outcomes vis-à-vis laparoscopic RBS (LRBS).

■ INDICATIONS OF REOPERATIVE BARIATRIC SURGERY

Due to the complex nature of reoperation, it is of utmost importance to understand the indication for the same and can be broadly classified as either due to failure or complications arising out of index bariatric procedure.

Failure of Index Bariatric Procedure

Insufficient Weight Loss

Different authors have used different criteria in the past to define adequate weight loss leading to a lack of consensus. As per the Adelaide study group, an excess weight loss (EWL) >50%, as previously described by Reinhold was considered sufficient, while Fobi et al. described an EWL <40% as failure of index operation.[11,12]

Weight Regain

Several definitions have been used to quantify weight regain depending on the parameter employed. An increase of >10 kg absolute weight or >25% EWL or body mass index (BMI) of >5 kg/m^2 or >15% of total body weight from nadir or regain to a BMI >35 kg/m^2 after successful weight loss has been termed as "weight regain."[13-15]

Recurrence of Obesity-related Comorbidities

The comorbidities like diabetes mellitus, hypertension, dyslipidemia, obstructive sleep apnea (OSA), and gastroesophageal reflux disease (GERD) can be defined as per the standardized outcomes reporting of American Society for Metabolic and Bariatric Surgery (ASMBS) and their outcomes can be categorized as complete/partial remission, improvement, unchanged, recurrence, deteriorated, or de novo.[16]

Complications of Index Bariatric Procedure

Notwithstanding the early complications like hemorrhage, leak, gastrointestinal obstruction, perforation, band slippage, or internal hernia requiring immediate reoperation at times, the revisional surgeries are advised more frequently for late complications. Although, complications like stricture, stenosis, ulceration, GERD, and malnutrition are common to most bariatric procedures and can occur in varying proportions, the procedure-specific complications and the variety of reoperative surgical options available for failure as well as complications in the form of conversions, corrections, or reversals are illustrated in **Table 1**.[17]

■ PREOPERATIVE ASSESSMENT

With a mortality rate of around 2% after reoperative bariatric surgery compared to reported range of 0.1–1.1% after primary bariatric operation, a thorough multidisciplinary evaluation must be performed before committing to a revisional procedure.[18]

Due to the multifactorial nature of the failure of bariatric surgery, the preoperative evaluation mandates deliberation to identify the anatomical and functional or psychosocial causes of the failed or complicated index bariatric surgery, besides operative details of the primary procedure and should include the following:
- *Assessment of biochemical parameters:*
  - Complete hemogram
  - Renal and liver function test
  - Iron profile (serum iron, folate, ferritin, transferrin saturation, and vitamin B12)

TABLE 1: Indication, type, and options of RBS according to the index bariatric operation.

Index procedure	Indication	Type of RBS	Options of RBS
AGB	Weight regain/ inadequate weight loss/comorbidity recurrence	Conversion	• Conversion to SG • Conversion to RYGB • Conversion to BPD-DS
	Complications		
	Slippage	Correction/ reversal	• Band relocation • Band removal
	Erosion	Reversal	• Band removal
	Intolerance	Correction/ reversal	• Band relocation • Band removal
	Pouch dilation	Reversal	• Band removal
	Port complication	Correction	• Port inspection • Band removal
SG	Weight regain/ inadequate weight loss/comorbidity recurrence	Conversion/ revision	• Re-sleeve gastrectomy • Conversion to RYGB • Conversion to BPD-DS
	Complications		
	Stricture	Correction/ conversion	• Endoscopic dilation • Re-sleeve gastrectomy • Conversion to RYGB
	GERD	Correction	• Endoscopic treatment • Magnetic sphincter augmentation • Conversion to RYGB
	Fistula	Revision/ conversion	• Reinforcement of the staple line • Endoscopic management • Conversion to RYGB
	Dilation	Correction	• Re-sleeve gastrectomy
RYGB	Weight regain/ inadequate weight loss/comorbidity recurrence	Revision/ conversion	• Pouch and GJ redo • Conversion to distal RYGB • Conversion to BPD-DS
	Complications		
	Marginal ulcer	Revision/ conversion/ reversal	• GJ redo • Reversal

Contd...

Contd...

Index procedure	Indication	Type of RBS	Options of RBS
	Fistula	Correction	• Endoscopic management • Fistulectomy • Gastric remnant resection/trimming • Pouch/GJ redo
	Candy cane syndrome	Correction	• Candy cane resection • GJ redo
	Internal hernia	Correction	• Hernia reduction and closure of mesenteric spaces
	Pouch dilation/stenosis	Correction	• Endoscopic dilation • Pouch trimming • Pouch/GJ redo
	GJ anastomosis dilation/stenosis	Correction	• Endoscopic dilation • GJ redo
	Jejunojejunal anastomosis stenosis/stricture	Correction	• Jejunojejunal anastomosis redo
	Malnutrition	Reversal	• Reversal
OAGB	Weight regain/inadequate weight loss/comorbidity recurrence	Revision/conversion	• Pouch and GJ redo • Conversion to distal OAGB • Conversion to BPD-DS
	Complications		
	Marginal ulcer	Revision/conversion/reversal	• GJ redo • Reversal
	Fistula	Correction	• Endoscopic management • Fistulectomy • Gastric remnant resection/trimming • Pouch/GJ redo
	Pouch dilation/stenosis	Correction	• Endoscopic dilation • Pouch trimming • Pouch/GJ redo
	GJ anastomosis dilation/stenosis	Correction	• Endoscopic dilation • GJ redo
	Malnutrition	Reversal	• Reversal

(AGB: adjustable gastric banding; BPD-DS: biliopancreatic diversion with duodenal switch; GERD: gastroesophageal reflux disease; GJ: gastrojejunal; OAGB: one-anastomosis gastric bypass; RBS: revisional bariatric surgery; RYGB: Roux-en-Y gastric bypass; SG: sleeve gastrectomy)

- Diabetic profile (blood sugars, fasting/postprandial; and if deranged-HbA1c, fasting insulin, and C-peptide)
    - Bone profile (serum calcium, phosphate, vitamin D3, and parathyroid hormone)
    - Endocrine evaluation (thyroid disorders, Cushing's syndrome, etc.)
- Ultrasonography abdomen to evaluate the status of liver and to rule out biliary pathology. Additionally, transient hepatic elastography (fibroscan) can be done to measure liver steatosis and fibrosis.
- Contrast upper gastrointestinal (UGI) study to delineate the anatomy and functional assessment of reflux.
- UGI endoscopy to identify sequelae of GERD such as esophagitis and Barrett's esophagus, besides hiatal hernia, marginal ulcer, stricture, stenosis, gastrogastric fistula, band erosions, dilated sleeve, or fundus.
- Cardiopulmonary evaluation to assess the performance status and optimize these patients in anticipation of a prolonged operative duration [electrocardiogram, 2D-echocardiography, lipid profile, serum homocysteine, blood gas analysis, chest X-ray, pulmonary function tests, and polysomnography (in presence of clinical suspicion of OSA)].
- Dietary and nutritional assessment to rule out inappropriate dietary habits.
- Psychological and behavioral assessment to rule out substance abuse, binge eating disorders, and personality and lifestyle disorders.
- *Optional investigations may be required depending on the patient's symptoms:*
    - *Computed tomography (CT) scan/CT volumetry:* Useful in defining the anatomical aberration detected on UGI contrast study, besides additional information on volume of sleeve or pouch can be retrieved.
    - *24-hour pH monitoring:* For objective evaluation of acid and nonacid reflux in patients with GERD.
    - *High-resolution manometry (HRM):* Helpful in patients with dysphagia in absence of any mechanical cause.
    - *Gastric emptying studies:* May be beneficial in patients with poor oral tolerance, nausea, and vomiting, especially after SG.

Preoperative Patient Counseling and Education

All patients undergoing evaluation for reoperative bariatric surgery must be counseled and educated in detail along with their immediate family members. They should be made part of the decision-making process in deciding the choice of the procedure, listing the several pros and cons of each option available, thereby helping the treating team in understanding and meeting patient's expectations. Moreover, the additional risks of postoperative complications with reoperative bariatric surgery like bleeding, leak, thrombotic events, etc. and postoperative dietary plans should be reaffirmed in this counseling.

■ REOPERATIVE BARIATRIC SURGERY

The very thought of operating again on the same structure will alert any operating surgeon on the possibility of higher postoperative complications. These concerns are even more profound in RBS, especially if the intervention is being performed for an acute complication like leak or bleeding or in patients with significant weight regain or insufficient weight loss. Majority of the studies comparing the primary versus RBS are retrospective in nature; however, they report expected outcomes in the form of higher perioperative complications with RBS. In the study by Howell et al., a significant difference in morbidity rate of 3.9 versus 14.8% in primary versus RBS was reported, whereas Deylgat et al. found a similar morbidity and length of stay (LOS), however with higher intraoperative complications such as serosal tearing, bleeding, and suture dehiscence in revisional RYGB patients (11.11 vs. 3.22%) compared to primary.[18,19] In another study by Zhang et al., comparing 172 patients of revisional RYGB with 172 paired primary RYGB patients, higher blood loss (463.7 vs. 113.3 mL), longer operative time (272.5 vs. 175.5 min) and LOS (5.6 vs. 2.5 days) were observed during revisional procedures.[20] Despite higher complications including increased reoperation rates (10.8 vs. 5.4%), patients who had undergone RBS experienced a significant improvement in BMI (44.7 ± 9.5 to 33.8 ± 7.5) and achieved 61.2% EWL.[21] In a recent study by Zafar et al., reporting predictors and consequences from a dataset of 43,280 patients who had undergone RYGB under the Metabolic and Bariatric Surgery Accreditation and Quality Improvement Program (MBSAQIP), the incidence of postoperative bleeding (POB) was 1.51% in primary RYGB compared to 2.4% in revisional RYGB.[22] In a multicenter trial, longer operative times (203 vs. 154 min, $p < 0.001$), increased number of readmissions for oral intolerance (10.5 vs. 6.7%, $p = 0.046$), and higher rates of gastrojejunal anastomosis stricture (6.4 vs. 2.7%, $p = 0.013$) were reported during revisional robot-assisted RYGB. However, there were no significant differences in overall and severe complications, anastomotic leak, conversion, or reoperation rates.[23] In another study from a high-volume center evaluating the outcomes of RRBS, the major morbidity and mortality rates reported were 3.9 and 1.3%, respectively. In this retrospective analysis, patients achieved an additional %EWL of 38.2% at 2 years with better weight loss outcomes in patients with weight loss failure as the indication for RBS.[24] Similar %EWL (60.7%) at 2 years was reported by another study in patients undergoing revisional robot-assisted RYGB, however, in a much smaller cohort of patients with weight loss failure.[25]

With revisional bariatric interventions becoming safer with time and expertise, the slightly higher morbidity can be deemed acceptable considering the weight loss achieved, resolution of comorbidities, and overall long-term benefits.

■ SURGICAL APPROACH

Despite the technical complexity associated with reoperative surgery, minimal access approach via laparoscopy has scored over the open approach. With the advancement in instrumentation and increase in expertise, the laparoscopic approach has delivered clear benefits of reduced blood loss, shorter LOS, improved recovery time, decreased wound infection, postoperative pain, and a significantly low incidence of the incisional hernia, even with the RBS.[26] With advantages of conventional laparoscopy well acknowledged, its technical drawbacks such as two-dimensional vision, lack of tactile feedback, counterintuitive movement, and instruments with limited degrees of freedom are considerable limitations. These become more challenging in bariatric procedures due to the additional anatomical complexities of patients with morbid obesity like hepatomegaly, intraperitoneal adiposity, and thick abdominal walls requiring large amounts of torque in making precise maneuvers such as intracorporeal suturing. Difficult anatomy, male gender, and higher BMI have also been associated with higher rates of complications such as leaks and mortality.[27] Notwithstanding the above drawbacks, conventional laparoscopy has established itself as the standard of care owing to its benefits and cost-effectiveness; however, some authors differ and advocated that a robotic approach could have more beneficial results, especially in complex revisional procedures.[28]

Laparoscopic versus Robot-assisted Revisional Bariatric Surgery

As results favoring one over the other approach remain inconclusive, a review of some of the recently published studies comparing the two approaches might provide some insight into their pros and cons. As per the literature, conversion to RYGB was the most frequently performed revisional procedure either for insufficient weight loss/weight regain or as a corrective measure of the complication arising out of primary bariatric procedure. One of the earliest studies comparing the two approaches in a nonrandomized fashion found increased postoperative surgical complications rate (13 vs. 1%) and longer hospitalization with robotic RYGB, however with a significantly less operative time.[29] The major drawbacks of robotic approach, in general, have been the higher costs and longer operative duration as reported by studies from Köckerling et al. and Acevedo et al. with no significant differences in the outcomes when comparing with laparoscopic approach.[30,31] In contrast, trials by Beckmann et al. and Lainas et al. observed a shorter operative time with a robot-assisted versus laparoscopic approach for primary RYGB. The two studies also found either lower or similar postoperative complications and comparable weight loss outcomes with robotic approach, respectively.[32,33] Moreover, Acevedo and colleagues observed that robotic approach was associated with less morbidity and mortality in primary RYGB compared to SG, thereby failing to establish a clear benefit of robotic approach in SG as well as its cost-effectiveness.[31]

Iranmanesh et al. reported overall comparable findings between patients undergoing robot-assisted laparoscopic primary RYGB (n = 806) and revisional RYGB (n = 266). Although the study was underpowered to detect differences, they observed that the complication rates with robot-assisted RBS remains below the reported morbidity associated with LRBS. This improvement could be attributed to the robotic assistance and might help in decreasing the morbidity levels of revisional surgeries to that of the primary procedures.[23] In a retrospective study from Moon et al., no statistically significant differences were noted between laparoscopic and robotic approaches in terms of LOS, 30-day readmission or reoperation rates. However, they observed that surgeons preferred the robot-assisted approach for complex conversion procedures such as RYGB to BPD-DS or RYGB to SG, whereas the most performed laparoscopic RBS was that of revision gastrojejunostomy.[34] In a systematic review evaluating the reasons for RBS, reporting of higher postoperative complication rates ranging from 0–39.3% in laparoscopic revisional surgeries has favored the robot-assisted approach.[35] However, the latest meta-analysis comprising of six studies with 29,890 patients (2,459 in robotic group) comparing the perioperative outcomes of RRBS versus LRBS found no difference in postoperative complications (RR 1.07, p = 0.9), conversions to open (RR 1.33, p = 0.3), LOS (SMD 0.04, p = 0.8), or operative time (RR 0.21, p = 0.5). Although, the review showed no significant benefit of RRBS, the authors stressed upon the need for high-quality studies to further investigate RRBS.[36]

■ ROBOT-ASSISTED REVISIONAL BARIATRIC SURGERY

As discussed earlier in this chapter, the role of robotic assistance in RBS is debatable as far as perioperative outcomes are concerned; however, it has its technical advantages in complex procedures. With more evidence coming in, these advantages may translate into significantly improved postoperative outcomes. Robotic assistance is already a preferred approach of many surgeons for complex RBS, not only for its technical ease but more importantly because of its short learning curve.

Learning Curve

Among all the standard bariatric procedures being performed today, laparoscopic RYGB is arguably the most difficult and challenging to perform, requiring a great deal of competency, training, and dexterity.[37] Earlier the learning curve for a RYGB was around 75–100 cases.[38,39] However, in view of the fact that lesser number of RYGB are being performed across the globe leading to inadequate exposure of the trainees, ASMBS has decreased the number of cases required for certification in bariatric surgery from 100 to 50. In contrast, the use of robotic assistance which mimics human hand motions, the learning curve for RRYGB has been drastically shortened by 90% to approximately ten cases.[40,41] Several studies have confirmed this significant improvement in the learning curve with reporting of comparable outcomes like mortality (<1%), conversion to open (1–3%), major morbidity rates (<5%), leak rate (<2%), and operative duration being equal to laparoscopic approach.[39,42,43-46]

Operating Room Set-up

Operating room larger than usual laparoscopic rooms are preferred for robotic platform to allow its proper storage and comfortable movement of operating room personnel. The room should preferably be a dedicated room with integrated systems for lighting, CO_2 insufflation, electrosurgical units, and anesthesia equipment. A schematic representation of operating room set-up has been depicted in **Figure 1**, although it may vary depending upon the size and space considerations of other operating rooms.

Patient Positioning

The patient is positioned supine on a specialized operating table that can accommodate the bariatric patients. The table must support the capacity of patients with super-obesity even in steep reverse Trendelenburg position at

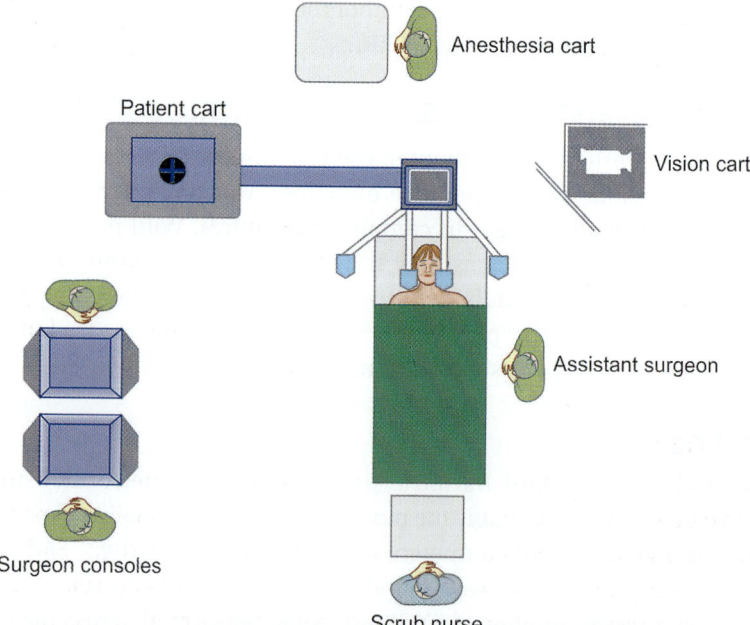

Fig. 1: Operating room set-up.

different heights as per the surgeon's preference to achieve the best exposure of the operative field. The patient is properly secured using safety straps with arms, lower waist, and legs properly tucked and padded. Pneumatic compression devices are applied over compression stockings on the lower limbs prior to the induction of anesthesia.

Port Placement

The port placement described is specific to the da Vinci Xi robotic system **(Fig. 2)**. The 12-mm camera port is placed in the periumbilical region, just to the left of the midline and CO_2 insufflation is kept at 15 mm Hg. Nathanson's retractor is then placed at epigastrium via 5 mm incision to retract the left lobe of liver out of the operative field. This was followed by the placement of 12-mm right mid-clavicular port, around one palm width below the right costal margin for introduction of stapling devices. Two 12-mm ports, one for table assistant and one working port for the surgeon, are placed at the level of camera port on either side of it. Finally, an 8-mm robotic assistant port is placed in left anterior axillary line. The surgical cart is then docked in position either from the patient's right or left side, and the arms attached to the four specific trocars.

Technical Advantages

The master-slave configuration with digital interface of robotic systems has outlined the fact that the robot's role is not to replace the surgeon but to help them perform complex tasks with more accuracy and more precision than standard laparoscopy.[47] One of the major early benefits of robotic assistance was the improved visualization in the form of stereoscopic 3D vision.[47,48] Robotic systems eliminate or filter the physiological tremor by downscaling the amplitude of the surgeon's motions by a factor of five or three to one,

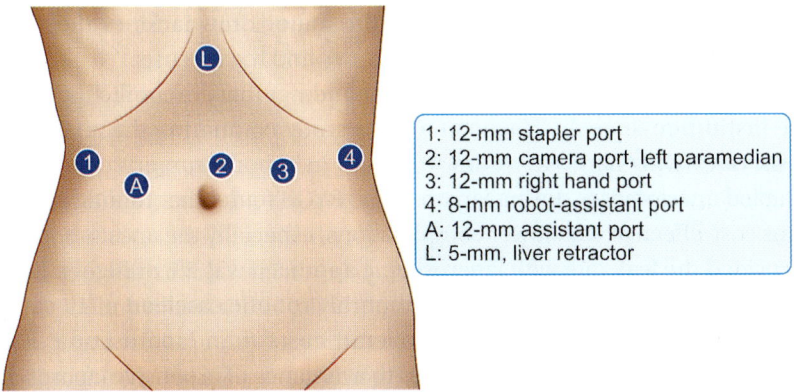

Fig. 2: Schematic diagram of usual port placement in robot-assisted revisional bariatric surgery (RRBS).

thereby increasing precision and stabilization.[49,50] Moreover, an additional seven degrees of freedom of movement provides wrist-like range of motion leading to enhanced manipulation of the tissue.[49] The additional movement at wrist of the robotic arm overcomes the torque encountered with thick abdominal walls of patients with obesity, a limitation which is characteristic of the standard laparoscopic approach and can lead to imprecise movements and surgeon fatigue.[48] The limitation of single quadrant surgery with earlier models of robotic platforms has been initially resolved with hybrid techniques using a combination of laparoscopy and robot. As several abdominal procedures including the bariatric surgery may require intervention in more than one quadrant of the abdomen, the advancements of the new da Vinci Xi System by Intuitive Surgical (Sunnyvale, CA, USA) has mitigated these concerns. Studies using a single dock, multiquadrant strategy for a successful conversion of adjustable gastric band to totally robotic BPD-DS and mobilization of colon with concomitant pelvic surgery in colorectal surgery have already been reported.[51,52] The benefits of robotic approach extend to the surgeons as conventional laparoscopic intervention has its concerns of poor ergonomics and incidences of surgeons reporting excessive fatigue and career-shortening musculoskeletal injuries due to prolonged operative duration in unnatural and sometimes awkward postures.[48-50,53-55] In contrast, the robotic platform offers a more natural posture with comfortable seating and more importantly, decreases the strain on the surgeon's shoulders, neck, and back muscles by using the robotic arms to overcome the abdominal wall torque.[50,56] The surgeons operating on robotic platforms have been able to perform difficult dissection and complex maneuvers including hand-sewn anastomoses at narrow spaces with fewer challenges and more freedom of movement, thereby prolonging their career.[48]

Drawbacks

Although few but near unanimous, the major drawbacks of the robotic platforms are the prolonged operative times and higher costs.

Studies reporting on cost-factor have findings that are conflicting and can be institution-specific. Hagen et al. in a study comparing the anastomotic leak rates with hand-sewn anastomoses in robotic surgery compared to stapled anastomoses during laparoscopic RYGB found that robotic approach was cost-effective with lower complications, especially the anastomotic leak, provided the leak rate with laparoscopic approach was 2% or higher. Further analysis in this trial showed that a monthly robotic caseload of 10 cases or more was associated with lower overall costs than laparoscopic RYGB, attributing the balancing of expenses to avoidance of expensive laparoscopic stapling devices.[42] Similar findings of lower costs with robotic approach have been documented by Rebecchi and team due to decreased use of staplers, improved operative duration with expertise, and lower maintenance cost with multidisciplinary use.[57]

Another uncommonly reported drawback of the robotic platforms was the relatively difficult and time-consuming process of removing the instruments and redocking the platform in procedures requiring changes in patient positioning.[28] This disadvantage has been alleviated with newer advances in robotic platforms making multiquadrant abdominal procedures feasible; however, procedures involving major positional changes during different steps of the surgery may still have this drawback. In addition, the literature on the role of the robot assistance in surgical emergencies is limited and remains under investigation.[58]

■ CONCLUSION

As a result of the advantages to the surgical team with its improved ergonomics, better dexterity and short learning curve, the potential of robotic assistance in RBS with its perioperative outcomes comparable to the conventional laparoscopy seems promising. The disadvantages of the higher costs and increased operative time are expected to become less evident with more widespread use, competing market brands, technical advancements of robotic platforms, and the availability of high-quality evidence in near future.

■ REFERENCES

1. English WJ, DeMaria EJ, Brethauer SA, Mattar SG, Rosenthal RJ, Morton JM. American Society for Metabolic and Bariatric Surgery estimation of metabolic and bariatric procedures performed in the United States in 2016. Surg Obes Relat Dis. 2018;14(3):259-63.
2. Altieri MS, Yang J, Nie L, Blackstone R, Spaniolas K, Pryor A. Rate of revisions or conversion after bariatric surgery over 10 years in the state of New York. Surg Obes Relat Dis. 2018;14(4):500-7.
3. Himpens J. Long-term outcomes of laparoscopic adjustable gastric banding. Arch Surg. 2011;146(7):802.
4. Van Gemert WG, Van Wersch MM, Greve JWM, Soeters PB. Revisional surgery after failed vertical banded gastroplasty: restoration of vertical banded gastroplasty or conversion to gastric bypass. Obes Surg. 1998;8:21-8.
5. Edholm D, Svensson F, Näslund I, Karlsson FA, Rask E, Sundbom M. Long-term results 11 years after primary gastric bypass in 384 patients. Surg Obes Relat Dis. 2013;9(5):708-13.
6. Colquitt JL, Pickett K, Loveman E, Frampton GK. Surgery for weight loss in adults. Cochrane Database Syst Rev. 2014;2014(8):1-16.
7. Gagner M. Laparoscopic revisional surgery after malabsorptive procedures in bariatric surgery, more specifically after duodenal switch. Surg Laparosc Endosc Percutan Tech. 2010;20(5):344-7.
8. Clapp B, Liggett E, Jones R, Lodeiro C, Dodoo C, Tyroch A. Comparison of robotic revisional weight loss surgery and laparoscopic revisional weight loss surgery using the MBSAQIP database. Surg Obes Relat Dis. 2019;15(6):909-99.

9. Horgan S, Vanuno D. Robots in laparoscopic surgery. J Laparoendosc Adv Surg Tech A. 2001;11(6):415-9.
10. Cheng YL, Elli EF. Role of robotic surgery in complex revisional bariatric procedures. Obes Surg. 2021;31:2583-9.
11. Hall J, Watts J, O'Brien P, Dunstan R, Walsh J, Slavotinek A, et al. Gastric surgery for morbid obesity–the Adelaide study. Amn Surg. 1990;211(4):419-27.
12. Fobi MAL, Lee H, Igwe D, Felahy B, James E, Stanczyk M, et al. Revision of failed gastric bypass to distal Roux-en-Y gastric bypass: a review of 65 cases. Obes Surg. 2001;11(2):190-5.
13. Lauti M, Lemanu D, Zeng ISL, Su'a B, Hill AG, MacCormick AD, et al. Definition determines weight regain outcomes after sleeve gastrectomy. Surg Obes Relat Dis. 2017;13(7):1123-9.
14. Nedelcu M, Khwaja HA, Rogula TG. Weight regain after bariatric surgery—how should it be defined? Surg Obes Relat Dis. 2016;12(5):1129-30.
15. Voorwinde V, Steenhuis IHM, Janssen IMC, Monpellier VM, van Stralen MM. Definitions of long-term weight regain and their associations with clinical outcomes. Obes Surg. 2020;30(2):527-36.
16. Brethauer SA, Kim J, el Chaar M, Papasavas P, Eisenberg D, Rogers A, et al. Standardized outcomes reporting in metabolic and bariatric surgery. Surg Obes Relat Dis. 2015;11(3):489-506.
17. Vanetta C, Dreifuss NH, Schlottmann F, Mangano A, Cubisino A, Valle V, et al. Current status of robot-assisted revisional bariatric surgery. J Clin Med. 2022;11(7):1820.
18. Howell RS, Liu HH, Boinpally H, Akerman M, Carruthers E, Brathwaite BM, et al. Outcomes of bariatric surgery: patients with body mass index 60 or greater. JSLS. 2021;25(2):e2020.00089.
19. Deylgat B, D'Hondt M, Pottel H, Vansteenkiste F, Van Rooy F, Devriendt D. Indications, safety, and feasibility of conversion of failed bariatric surgery to Roux-en-Y gastric bypass: a retrospective comparative study with primary laparoscopic Roux-en-Y gastric bypass. Surg Endosc. 2012;26(7): 1997-2002.
20. Zhang L, Tan WH, Chang R, Eagon JC. Perioperative risk and complications of revisional bariatric surgery compared to primary Roux-en-Y gastric bypass. Surg Endosc. 2015;29:1316-20.
21. Fulton C, Sheppard C, Birch D, Karmali S, de Gara C. A comparison of revisional and primary bariatric surgery. Can J Surg. 2017;60:205-11.
22. Zafar SN, Miller K, Felton J, Wise ES, Kligman M. Postoperative bleeding after laparoscopic Roux en Y gastric bypass: predictors and consequences. Surg Endosc. 2019;33(1):272-80.
23. Iranmanesh P, Fam J, Nguyen T, Talarico D, Chandwani KD, Bajwa KS, et al. Outcomes of primary versus revisional robotically assisted laparoscopic Roux-en-Y gastric bypass: A multicenter analysis of ten-year experience. Surg Endosc. 2021;35:5766-73.
24. Dreifuss NH, Mangano A, Hassan C, Masrur MA. Robotic revisional bariatric surgery: a high-volume center experience. Obes Surg. 2021;31(4):1656-63.
25. Bindal V, Gonzalez-Heredia R, Elli EF. Outcomes of robot-assisted roux-en-y gastric bypass as a reoperative bariatric procedure. Obes Surg. 2015;25(10): 1810-5.

26. Mun EC, Blackburn GL, Matthews JB. Current status of medical and surgical therapy for obesity. Gastroenterology. 2001;120(3):669-81.
27. Fazylov RM, Savel RH, Horovitz JH, Pagala MK, Coppa GF, Nicastro J, et al. Association of super-super-obesity and male gender with elevated mortality in patients undergoing the duodenal switch procedure. Obes Surg. 2005;15(5):618-23.
28. Giulianotti PC, Coratti A, Angelini M, Sbrana F, Cecconi S, Balestracci T, et al. Robotics in general surgery: Personal experience in a large community hospital. Arch Surg. 2003;138:777-84.
29. Benizri EI, Renaud M, Reibel N, Germain A, Ziegler O, Zarnegar R, et al. Perioperative outcomes after totally robotic gastric bypass: a prospective nonrandomized controlled study. Am J Surg. 2013;206:145-51.
30. Köckerling F. Robotic vs. standard laparoscopic technique-what is better? Front Surg. 2014;1:15.
31. Acevedo E, Mazzei M, Zhao H, Lu X, Soans R, Edwards MA. Outcomes in conventional laparoscopic versus robotic-assisted primary bariatric surgery: a retrospective, case–controlled study of the MBSAQIP database. Surg Endosc. 2020;34:1353-65.
32. Beckmann JH, Bernsmeier A, Kersebaum JN, Mehdorn AS, Taivankhuu T, Laudes M, et al. The impact of robotics in learning Roux-en-Y gastric bypass: a retrospective analysis of 214 laparoscopic and robotic procedures: robotic vs. laparoscopic RYGB. Obes Surg. 2020;30:2403-10.
33. Lainas P, Kassir R, Benois M, Derienne J, Debs T, Safieddine M, et al. Comparative analysis of robotic versus laparoscopic Roux-en-Y gastric bypass in severely obese patients. J Robot Surg. 2021;15(6):891-8.
34. Moon RC, Segura AR, Teixeira AF, Jawad MA. Feasibility and safety of robot-assisted bariatric conversions and revisions. Surg Obes Relat Dis. 2020;16:1080-5.
35. Pinto-Bastos A, Conceicao EM, Machado PPP. Reoperative bariatric surgery: a systematic review of the reasons for surgery, medical and weight loss outcomes, relevant behavioral factors. Obes Surg. 2017;27:2707-15.
36. Bertoni MV, Marengo M, Garofalo F, Volontè F, La Regina D, Gass M, et al. Robotic-Assisted versus laparoscopic revisional bariatric surgery: a systematic review and meta-analysis on perioperative outcomes. Obes Surg. 2021;31(11):5022-33.
37. Hubens G, Balliu L, Ruppert M, Gypen B, Van Tu T, Vaneerdeweg W. Roux-en-Y gastric bypass procedure performed with the da Vinci robot system: is it worth it? Surg Endosc. 2008;22(7):1690-6.
38. Schauer P, Ikramuddin S, Hamad G, Gourash W. The learning curve for laparoscopic Roux-en-Ygastric bypass is 100 cases. Surg Endosc. 2003;17(2):212-5.
39. Oliak D, Ballantyne GH, Weber P, Wasielewski A, Davies RJ, Schmidt HJ. Laparoscopic Roux-en-Y gastric bypass: defining the learning curve. Surg Endosc. 2003;17(3):405-8.
40. Mohr CJ, Nadzam GS, Curet MJ. Totally robotic Roux-en-Y gastric bypass. Arch Surg. 2005;140:779-86.
41. Sanchez BR, Mohr CJ, Morton JM, Safadi BY, Alami RS, Curet MJ. Comparison of totally robotic laparoscopic Roux-en-Y gastric bypass and traditional laparoscopic Roux-en-Y gastric bypass. Surg Obes Relat Dis. 2005;1(6):549-54.

42. Hagen ME, Pugin F, Chassot G, Huber O, Buchs N, Iranmanesh P, et al. Reducing cost of surgery by avoiding complications: the model of robotic Roux-en-Y gastric bypass. Obes Surg. 2012;22(1):52-61.
43. Higa KD, Boone KB, Ho T. Complications of the laparoscopic Roux-en-Y gastric bypass: 1,040 patients—what have we learned? Obes Surg. 2000;10(6):509-13.
44. Higa KD, Boone KB, Ho T, Davies OG. Laparoscopic Roux-en-Y gastric bypass for morbid obesity: technique and preliminary results of our first 400 patients. Arch Surg. 2000;135(9):1029-33, discussion 33-4.
45. Matthews BD, Sing RF, DeLegge MH, Ponsky JL, Heniford BT. Initial results with a stapled gastrojejunostomy for the laparoscopic isolated roux-en-Y gastric bypass. Am J Surg. 2000;179(6):476-81.
46. Nguyen NT, Goldman C, Rosenquist CJ, Arango A, Cole CJ, Lee SJ, et al. Laparoscopic versus open gastric bypass: a randomized study of outcomes, quality of life, and costs. Ann Surg. 2001;234(3):279-89, discussion 89-91.
47. Talamini MA, Chapman S, Horgan S, Melvin WS, Academic Robotics group. A prospective analysis of 211 robotic-assisted surgical procedures. Surg Endosc. 2003;17:1521-4.
48. Bindal V, Bhatia P, Dudeja U, Kalhan S, Khetan M, John S, et al. Review of contemporary role of robotics in bariatric surgery. J Minim Access Surg. 2015;11:16-21.
49. Cadière GB, Himpens J, Germay O, Izizaw R, Degueldre M, Bruyns J, et al. Feasibility of robotic laparoscopic surgery: 146 cases. World J Surg. 2001;25:1467-77.
50. Jara RD, Guerrón AD, Portenier D. Complications of robotic surgery. Surg Clin North Am. 2020;100:461-8.
51. Sudan R, Desai S. Conversion of laparoscopic adjustable gastric band to robot-assisted laparoscopic biliopancreatic diversion with duodenal switch. Surg Obes Relat Dis. 2011;7:546-7.
52. Protyniak B, Jorden J, Farmer R. Multiquadrant robotic colorectal surgery: the da Vinci Xi vs Si comparison. J Robot Surg. 2018;12:67-74.
53. Toro JP, Lin E, Patel AD. Review of robotics in foregut and bariatric surgery. Surg Endosc. 2015;29:1-8.
54. Esposito C, El Ghoneimi A, Yamataka A, Rothenberg S, Bailez M, Ferro M, et al. Work-related upper limb musculoskeletal disorders in paediatric laparoscopic surgery. A multicenter survey. J Pediatr Surg. 2013;48:1750-6.
55. Janki S, Mulder EEAP, IJzermans JNM, Khe Tran TC. Ergonomics in the operating room. Surg Endosc. 2017;31:2457-66.
56. Wilson EB, Sudan R. The evolution of robotic bariatric surgery. World J Surg. 2013;37:2756-60.
57. Rebecchi F, Ugliono E, Allaix ME, Toppino M, Borello A, Morino M. Robotic Roux-en-Y gastric bypass as a revisional bariatric procedure: a single-center prospective cohort study. Obes Surg. 2019;30(1):11-17.
58. de'Angelis N, Khan J, Marchegiani F, Bianchi G, Aisoni F, Alberti D, et al. Robotic surgery in emergency setting: 2021 WSES position paper. World J Emerg Surg. 2022;17:4

CHAPTER 14

Robotic Hysterectomy: How I do it? Sinha—Apollo Technique

Rooma Sinha, Bana Rupa, Mamtha Reddy

■ INTRODUCTION

Laparoscopic hysterectomy was first described in 1989 by Harry Reich.[1] Still abdominal approach remains the primary method in many centers.[2] In 2005, FDA approved for use of Da Vinci Robotic System in gynecology and since then, it has been used worldwide to perform minimal access hysterectomy. A new technology can often perplex surgeons and delay universal adoption in their surgical practice. We will discuss a "Sinha-Apollo Technique" for Da Vinci system in performing robotic-assisted laparoscopic hysterectomy (RALH) in simplified and reproducible steps. It is a two arms–three instruments technique.

■ SURGICAL PROCEDURE

Presurgical Preparation (Figs. 1 and 2)

The previous day patients take liquid diet and two tablets of bisacodyl in the night and arrive at the hospital on the day of their surgery. The operating table is lined with an antislip mattress and two folded bed sheets. Hands are secured in a sleeve to prevent dislodgement of intravenous line or pulse

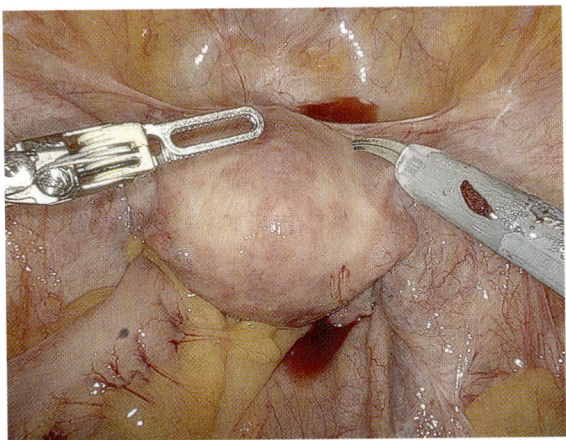

Fig. 1: Selection of instruments fenestrated bipolar hot shears and monopolar scissors.

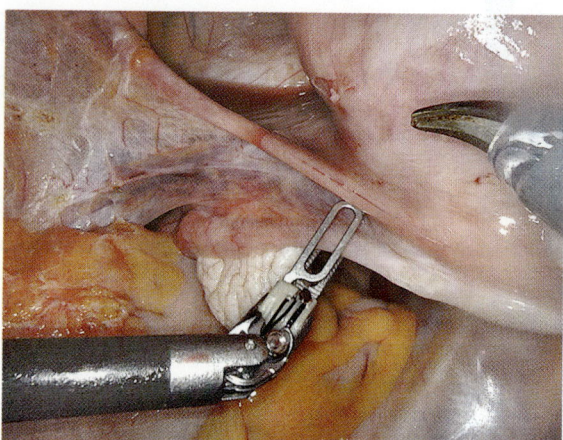

Fig. 2: Starting from left side ovarian ligament.

oximeter probe. The head is supported with a foam pillow and the face is covered with a folded bed sheet. The draw sheets are used as a brace to stabilize the patient, and hands tucked by the side with the palm facing toward the thigh and thumbs up. The patient is put in a modified dorsal lithotomy with hip flexion (120–170°), knee flexion (90–120°), externally rotated hip abduction (<90°). We use Rumi uterine manipulator system with Advincula Arch (CooperSurgical, Trumbull, CT, USA). An appropriate size of Rumi tip and Koh cup is selected. Efficient manipulation helps in avoiding the need for a third robotic arm. The beveled edge of the Koh cup identifies the trajectory of colpotomy. Bladder is drained intraoperatively with Foley's catheter.

Port Placement and Positioning

The primary optic port is placed with modified Hasson's technique. This is either placed at the umbilicus or at a supraumbilical position. The left and right robotic trocars (8 mm, Intuitive Surgical, Inc., Sunnyvale, CA, USA) are placed 8–10 cm lateral to midline and 3–4 cm inferior to the optic trocar. A line is then drawn from the left 8 mm trocar and the optic trocar. At the midpoint of this line a perpendicular line is drawn in the cranial direction and a 5 mm assistant port is placed 4–5 cm from the line **(Fig. 2)**.

Before docking, a survey of the abdominal cavity is done, and small bowel and sigmoid colon is displaced and tucked in the cephalic direction. The Trendelenburg position of 15–20 degrees tilt is done. Attention to the position is important as this cannot be changed once the patient cart is docked. The patient cart is placed on the side, parallel to the operating table, giving space between the legs for the use of uterine manipulator. Once targeting is done, the arms are docked on either side.

Surgical Steps

We use a 30-degree telescope for RALH and advocate a sequential strategy to complete all left side ligaments and uterine complex up to the colpotomy ring before moving to the right side. The ureters are identified and their path traced transperitoneally. Fenestrated bipolar in arm 3 (40 watts) and hot shear monopolar scissors is selected in arm 1 (30 watts) **(Fig. 1)**. The arm 2 has the telescope. We begin with the left round ligament and ovarian pedicle which are coagulated and transected **(Fig. 2)**. Salpingectomy and/or oophorectomy is done in the end after completion of the hysterectomy giving an unobstructed view of the broad ligament. The anterior leaf of broad ligament is opened using the hot shears and the dissection proceeds anteriorly to cut the vesico-uterine reflection and dissecting the bladder down **(Fig. 3)**. The posterior left leaf of broad ligament and the left uterosacral ligament are now coagulated and transected **(Fig. 4)**. This helps to skeletonize the left uterine artery and

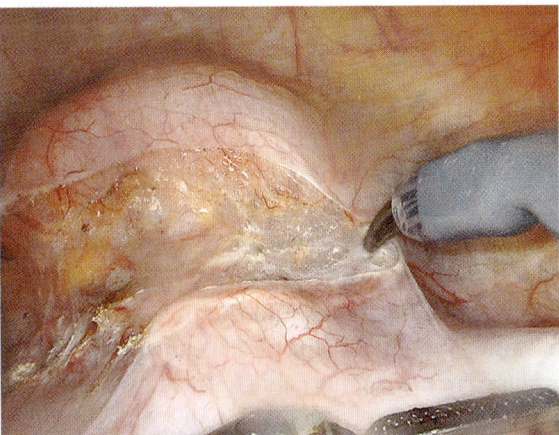

Fig. 3: Dissection of uterovesical fold of peritoneum.

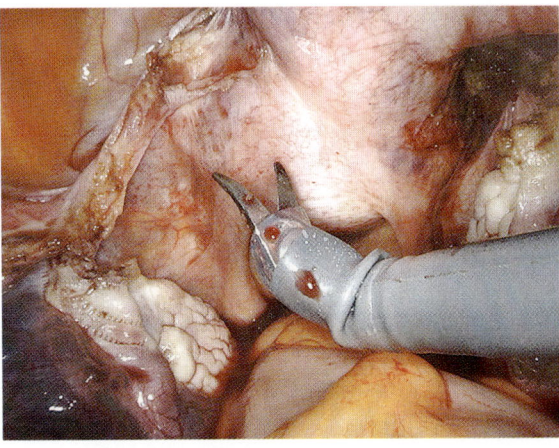

Fig. 4: Approach to uterosacral ligaments.

vein as it enters the uterus at the cervicouterine junction. The assistant then pushes the uterus in cephalad direction with the help of uterine manipulator delineating the Koh cup which is the ultimate destination of this side of dissection. This cephalad movement helps the ureters fall laterally and away from harm's way. Skeletonization of the uterine vessels and a tension-free application (slightly loose grip) of the bipolar forceps ensures adequate tissue effect and robust sealing of the vessels before transection and minimizing the lateral thermal spread. The uterine artery and vein is then coagulated and transected by a synchronized movement of fenestrated bipolar and hot shears. We describe this as the "Salsa maneuver" **(Fig. 5)**.

Coagulation of the ascending branches of the uterine vessels reduces back flow from the specimen. Once the left side pedicles are completed, we then move to the right sided pedicles and follow the same steps to reach up to the Koh cup (colpotomy ring). After coagulation of bilateral uterine vessels, the uterus appears blanched and the colpotomy is then begun from the anterior vaginal vault. Monopolar hot shears is used to divide the cardinal ligament complexes of the left side first and then the right side in a manner consistent with an intrafascial hysterectomy. The camera is then flipped with 30 degrees up and the posterior part of colpotomy is completed. At this stage the pneumoperitoneum is maintained by inflation of the pneumo-occluder balloon and placed in vagina. This is a sequential method to approach the vaginal vault **(Figs. 6A to D)**.

Removal of tubes and/or ovaries is done at this stage. After identification of the infundibulopelvic ligaments and the ureters, bipolar coagulation is done with fenestrated bipolar and the pedicle transected with the hot shears. The adnexa is placed in the vaginal canal for retrieval **(Fig. 7)**. The specimen along within the adnexa is retrieved vaginally with or with morcellation. Morcellation if needed is done with a scalpel with number 11 blade. Repeated

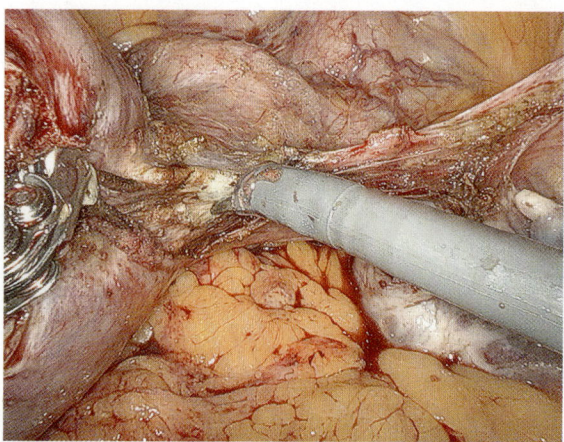

Fig. 5: Uterine artery coagulation transection: The Salsa technique.

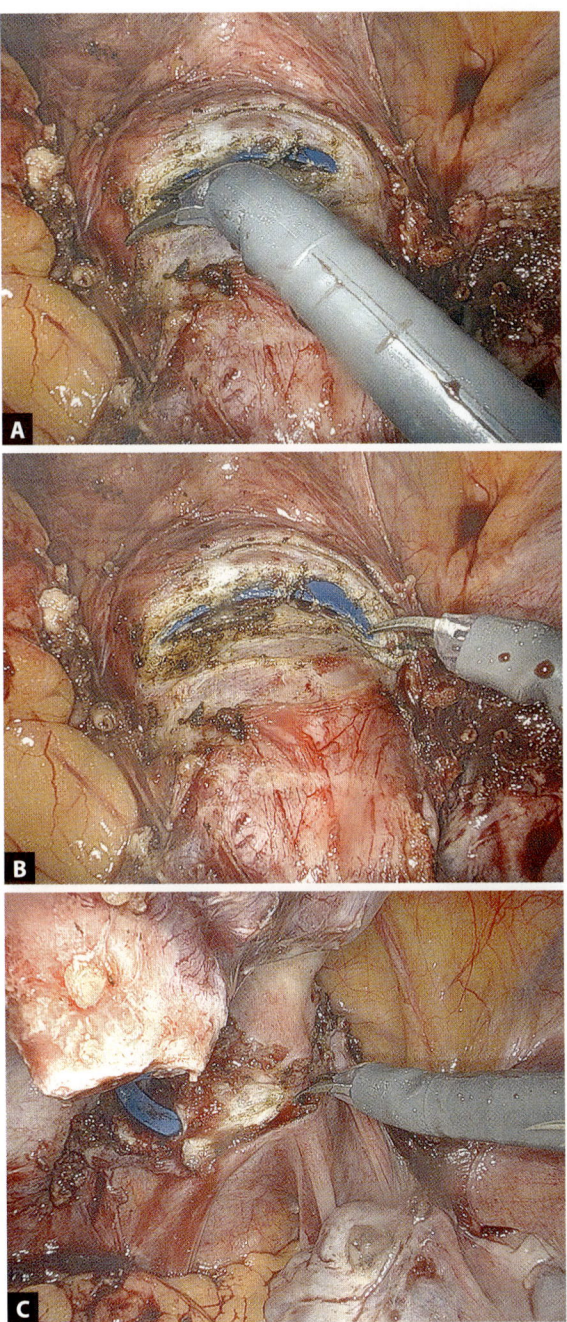

Figs. 6A to C: *Contd...*

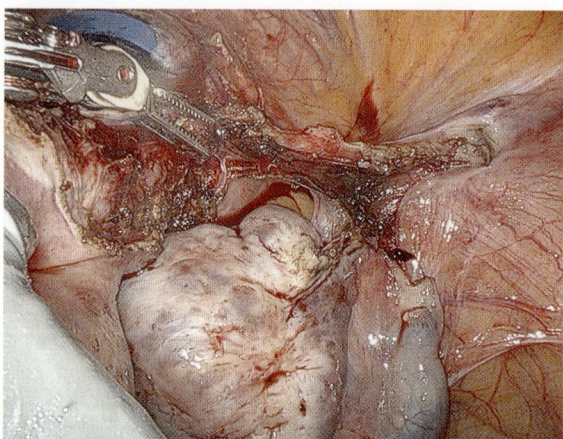

Fig. 6D

Figs. 6A to D: (A) Anterior colpotomy; (B) Complete anterior colpotomy; (C) Extending colpotomy incision posteriorly; (D) Approach of colpotomy at the right vaginal vault angle.

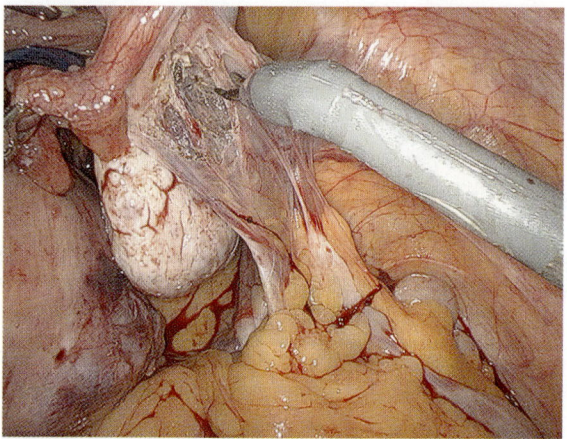

Fig. 7: Removal of adnexa in the end.

curved linear incisions are made in order to make a globular uterine specimen into a longitudinal one and removed vaginally. We use umbilical port for morcellation if the vagina is very narrow after containing uterus in a bag. The vaginal cuff closure is accomplished with the fenestrated forceps in arm 3 which is used to grasp and evert the edges of the vaginal cuff and a mega needle driver in arm 1. Using a 5 × 5 rule, each vaginal bite is taken at a distance of 5 mm and for a depth of 5 mm on the cut edge including both the vaginal fascia and vaginal epithelium in each bite **(Fig. 8)**. This ensures robust closure of the vault reducing the postoperative dehiscence. Adequate hemostasis at the vault reduces the incidence of postoperative hematoma but

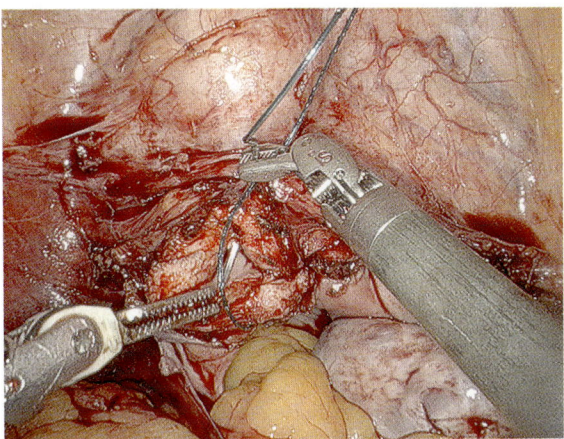

Fig. 8: Vaginal vault suturing using the 5 × 5 rule.

an overzealous cauterization should be avoided. A 15 cm 1-0 V-Loc barbed suture (Medtronic, Minneapolis, MN, USA) on a GS21 needle is used. This closure is done in a single layer with the inclusion of the uterosacral ligament to prevent future vault prolapse. The end of the barbed suture is cut flush with vault and the needle retrieved.

Prior to closure, all operative sites are irrigated, a low insufflation pressure check is performed to ensure hemostasis, and the patient cart is undocked after removing all instruments. Ports are removed under vision. The pneumoperitoneum is released in the smoke evacuation system. The rectus sheath of the primary port is identified at the umbilicus and closed with number 1/0 polypropylene. The rectus sheath of the 8 mm ports is not routinely closed. All port skin is closed with number 3/0 poliglecaprone absorbable suture.

■ DISCUSSION

The RALH described by Advincula in 2006 used three operative ports and five robotic instruments.[3] We began doing RALH by the same method in 2012, however realized after about 25 cases that we can reduce the number of ports as well as instruments used during the surgery. We reduced the ports to only two operative ports and use only fenestrated bipolar and hot shears to perform the hysterectomy. The original technique described placement of surgical cart between the patient's legs but we place it on the right side of the patient parallel to the operating table giving ample room for efficient uterine manipulation by the assistant. We modified the assistant trocar from 11 to 5 mm and also started placing them on the left side above the 8 mm trocar as described in our procedure. In the initial procedure description, steep Trendelenburg was used. We do not use "steep" Trendelenburg as lower angles are effective during gynecological robotic procedures.[4] During the vault closure we used a mega needle driver in arm 1 and continued to use the fenestrated bipolar in arm 2 to suture the vault with V-Loc suture. Few modifications mentioned here have also been adopted by same authors in their subsequent publication.[5]

■ CONCLUSION

Despite improvements in endoscopic technology, laparoscopic hysterectomy is not universally adopted. Simple and reproducible steps described as the Sinha-Apollo Technique can reduce the learning curve and increase the adoption of RALH. The use of two arms and three instruments translates in cost reduction. The strategy of completing the surgical steps on one side up to the colpotomy cup before moving to the other side enhances the economy of movements and makes the whole surgery time efficient.

■ REFERENCES

1. Reich H, DeCaprio J, McGlynn F. Laparoscopic Hysterectomy. J Gynecol Surg. 1989;5(2):213-6.
2. Cohen SL, Vitonis AF, Einarsson JI. Updated hysterectomy surveillance and factors associated with minimally invasive hysterectomy. J Soc Laparoendosc Surg. 2014;18(3):e2014.00096.
3. Advincula AP. Surgical techniques: Robot-assisted laparoscopic hysterectomy with the da Vinci® surgical system. Int J Med Robot Comput Assist Surg. 2006;2(4):305-11.
4. Ghomi A, Kramer C, Askari R, Chavan NR, Einarsson JI. Trendelenburg position in gynecologic robotic-assisted surgery. J Minim Invasive Gynecol. 2012;19(4):485-9.
5. Simpson KM, Advincula AP. The essential elements of a robotic-assisted laparoscopic hysterectomy. Obstet Gynecol Clin North Am. 2016;43:479-93.

CHAPTER 15

Biomimetics and Artificial Intelligence: Pushing the Frontiers of Robotic Surgery

Shyamanta M Hazarika

Abstract

Technological advances, particularly in artificial intelligence (AI) and robotics, are being applied broadly in society and increasingly in healthcare including surgery. Surgery that has evolved over the ages, saw robotic interventions as early as 1980s. Despite its early initiation, robots in surgery could only make incremental advances; remained formative in spite of being an innovative disruption. However, with recent advances in AI and robotics together with progress in minimally invasive surgery (MIS), today robotic surgery seeks to evolve novel strategies of surgical interventions toward improved clinical outcomes. Biomimetic robotics and AI are pushing the frontiers of innovation in robotic surgery. AI is surging ahead; AI-powered biomimetic robots are poised to change the world of surgery in more ways than one could possibly imagine. This article discusses about the aspects of biomimetics and AI as they pertain to the modern practice of robotic surgery with a focus on current trends and future directions.

■ INTRODUCTION

Surgery has a long and chequered history. From a marked regression in surgical knowledge during the Middle Ages, the convergence to modern surgery is a story of multiple breakthroughs. Modern surgery has been made possible not only with the gain of anatomical and physiological knowledge but also tremendous advancement in enabling technologies such as anesthetics, antiseptics, antibiotics, and analgesics. Possibly the dream of approaches for scarless surgery, spearheaded the birth of minimally invasive surgery (MIS). Quest for diagnosis techniques not relying on open procedures together with the progress in medical imaging changed the face of modern surgery. Computers became an integral part of the team assisting the surgeon in performance of his task. An increasing demand for greater precision led to robotic interventions in surgery as early as 1980s; with the first surgical robot being developed based on an industrial robotic manipulator.[1] Despite its early initiation, robots in surgery could only make incremental advances; remained formative in spite of being an innovative disruption.

The earliest of the surgical robots in clinical practice was stereotaxic.[1] It required human surgical review on conclusion of each step of robotic surgery gravitating a master-slave architecture. Soft-tissue surgical capability and far-reaching advantages over traditional MIS led to the development of endoscopic robotic systems.[2] Ergonomics and visualization in robot assisted surgery (RAS) are far beyond traditional laparoscopy. Today robotic surgery seeks to evolve novel strategies of surgical interventions toward improved clinical outcomes through improved precision, smaller incision, and reduced trauma.[3]

Miniaturization is a major dimension of research in surgical robotics. As we make progress in our quest for precision, smaller-sized surgical robots minimizing collateral tissue damage and scarring are being conceived. Laparoendoscopic single-port surgery (LESS) and natural orifice transluminal endoscopic surgery (NOTES) have emerged as encouraging approaches of RAS. Robots engaged in such procedures need to perform in vivo manipulations and need to be miniaturized. MIS and endoscopic methodologies had long begun adopting bioinspired technologies for miniaturization. While LESS or NOTES seeks to improve on existing approaches, miniaturization driven through biomimicry is taking a completely different route through microbots for surgery. Microbots as the name suggests are submillimeter robots. These mobile robots with built-in surgical functionalities are possible to be deployed into a patient's bloodstream; controlled and maneuvered to a specific destination within the human anatomy to carry out a designated task.[4] AI-powered biomimetic microbots are poised to change the world of surgery in more ways than one could possibly imagine.

Recent advances in artificial intelligence (AI) and robotics, together with progress in medical imaging is changing the way modern surgery is performed. Multimodal data integration has made possible planning the surgery in virtual environment; three-dimensional (3D) mental reconstruction for diagnosis and planning may no longer be required. While the surgeon is coming to terms with planning in a virtual environment, a new dream is being woven. The primary thrust is shifting from augmenting the surgeon through the capabilities of a robot to emphasis on more autonomy to the robotic system, heading toward an autonomous surgical robot. Note that autonomy here refers to the ability to perform intended tasks without human intervention. Robotic surgeons powered through embodied cognition, possessing capability to take decisions and communicate effectively with the human counterpart will eventually find their way into the operation theatre of the future. As of today, a fully automated robotic surgical system remains conceptual. Nevertheless, there have been multiple recent developments toward accomplishing supervised robotic surgery systems with evident degrees of autonomy.[5] Autonomous systems are the future of AI. AI is surging ahead; pushing the frontiers of innovation in robotic surgery.

Over the last decade, robotic surgery has made substantial progress. It is a story of innovations coupled with technological improvements. This short article, rather than making an attempt to present an exhaustive review of the innovations and accomplishments in the field, is devoted to provide insights of two very important facets; biomimetics for robot development and autonomy through AI. There exist brilliant reviews on robotic surgery[2,3] including microbots for surgery.[4,6] This article discusses about aspects of biomimetics and AI as they pertain to the modern practice of robotic surgery, with a focus on current trends and future directions.

■ BIOMIMETIC INTERVENTIONS

Biomimetics or biomimicry is the study of nature's designs and processes in search of inspiration for creating efficient machines. The core idea is to imitate biological structures or behaviors, building in them a capability to adapt to the environment.[7] Biomimetics has emerged as a powerful tool to solve many complex problems including those in surgical robotics. Surgical robots looked for bioinspiration to produce instruments with articulated tips; creating artifacts that would allow access to hard-to-reach areas. Biomimicry together with multiple articulation created highly articulated endoscopes that resembled snakes, octopuses and similar flexible systems that could reconfigure itself and stiffen by actuation.[8]

Microbots and Biomimetics

In spite of being simple single-celled organisms at the micro-scale, micro-organisms possess machinery that empowers them to sense and act on their environment. Creation of artificial micro-robots and microscopic machines exhibiting behavioral sophistication of micro-organisms has been a long-cherished dream. Miniaturization is not straightforward; one cannot simply come down on the size of a traditional robot to the microscale creating a micro-robot. Rather, biomimetic design principles are followed to create a *replica*; often mimicking sensing, actuation and control, so as to have robotic functionalities. This enables microbots to accomplish specific tasks, either autonomously or semi-autonomously, making them the candidates of choice for minimally invasive medical interventions.[9]

Microrobotic procedures are in the forefront of RAS. Larger robotic systems with relatively inflexible structures, functioning through traditional surgical approaches is making away for microbots. Microbots are untethered systems; systems with no physical connection to a master console or an operator arm. Microbots could work alone or in groups, entering the human body with minimal surgical intervention. Capsule endoscopes a category of microbots are already in clinical use.[10] These microbots function predominantly as imaging modalities. Unlike microbots for robotic surgery, capsule endoscopes are passive; transported by the peristaltic motility of the gastrointestinal system. Microbots for surgery ranging from micro-grippers to micro-bullets need specialized components. Apart from imaging, control and communication, such microbots need to include contained propulsion for locomotion and miniaturized functionality for tissue manipulation. This is where advances in biomimicry come to the rescue.

Bioinspired propulsion: Microrobots for MIS spend most of its life navigating inside fluids. Autonomous locomotion could be based on as diverse organisms as a swimming micro-organism, a fish, or a snake. Salamanders provide inspiration of locomotion strategies optimized for two targeted districts, stomach and colon; the capsule swims in a liquid environment of the stomach and moves by legs in the colon. However, navigating inside a fluid in microscale is different from a macroscale robot swimming in a fluid. Viscous forces are far higher than the inertial forces acting on a microbot. Micro-organisms exploit appendages such as cilia and flagella to execute nonreciprocal propulsive movement. Take inspiration from such micro-organisms, appendages such as the cilia and flagella are mimicked in microbots for controlled propulsion.[11] Rotation of flagella, as seen in a bacterium, could lead to translational motion. Rather than any on-board micromotor for rotation, an external rotating magnetic field drives these micropropellers.

Biomimetic micro-instruments: Surgery microrobots are distinguishably different from other microbots. These microbots have on-board functional micro-instruments that allow performance of surgical maneuvers such as dissecting, grasping, and ablation. Bioinspired spring driven micro-spikes and vibrating micro-pipettes form the armory for cutting and dissection. Grasping and manipulation involves use of micro-grippers based on human appendages; a central palm from which multiple digits originate.[12] Diverse array of surgical procedures is feasible using microrobots. This could possibly be achieved with far less collateral damage to healthy tissue compared to state-of-the-art robotic surgery procedures.

Autonomous and collective behavior: Powered through biomimetics, microrobotics endeavors to design functional and autonomous microbots. Active matter refers to systems composed of self-driven units. This is being exploited to have autonomous motion and collective behavior showing equivalences to the organization of flocks of birds, schools of fishes or bacterial colonies. Chemically and externally driven active systems strive to equip next generation of microrobots with intelligence and eventually, autonomy advancing the field of microsurgery.[11]

Cyborgs: Is This the Future?

Taking bioinspiration to a different level, there have been attempts to take advantages of biological organisms by controlling their functionalities *per se*. Unlike traditional biomimetic approach, no attempt is made for electromechanical replication of their form and function. Controlled use of the biological organism involves exploiting the sensory organs for information exchange and musculoskeletal system for dexterous manipulation. Growing interest in cybernetics and rapid progression of micro-electro-mechanical systems (MEMS) have created possibilities of building cyborgs, hybrid systems that incorporate artificial and biological elements in a single entity.[6] Major challenge in use of such hybrid systems lies in the ability to effectively regulate the system. Thermal microstimulation has been reported to be effective for control of locomotion. Traditional sterilization methods will not work for hybrid systems; in vivo use and control of cyborgs remains a major challenge.

■ ARTIFICIAL INTELLIGENCE AND SURGICAL ROBOTICS

To be intelligent, robots need to have abilities to sense-plan-act. The sense-plan-act cycle is what endows it the capability to undertake tasks "automatically", either programmed or autonomously. Almost all of the current robotic platforms are nowhere near; most of these machines lack the ability to independently sense, plan, and act. AI would bring with it the ability to learn and take decisions, making the surgical robots autonomous. AI is aimed at enhancing the capabilities of surgical robotic systems. This could include improvements in perception, localization and mapping of complex in vivo environment; resourceful decision-making; and performing required tasks with improved precision, safety, and efficiency.

Facets of Artificial Intelligence in Robotic Surgery

Artificial intelligence is demonstrated when any task, formerly performed by a human and thought of as requiring the ability to learn, reason and solve problems, can be done by a machine. Intelligence requires knowledge. Knowledge is accrued through a process of learning. Machine learning (ML) focuses on the ability of machines to receive data and extract patterns or making meaning out of the data. This is what makes the role of ML significant in our quest to create intelligent surgical robots.

Artificial intelligence in robotic surgery has strong roots in imaging and visualization. With AI-powered functions, real-time sensing offers the possibility of robotic control. With varying levels of autonomy, the surgical robot and the surgeon can create synergy to navigate and operate in vivo.

Learning from demonstration: Deep learning including deep neural networks are ML approaches exploiting data for learning rather than understanding task specific algorithms. From huge repository of data, ML techniques allow surgical robots to have critical insights and state-of-art practices. These insights are productively shared with surgeon; while the robot is made to learn from demonstrations. Imitation learning or learning from demonstration (LfD) enables a robot to perform autonomously new tasks with learned policies.[13] LfD involves segmentation of a complex task into several motion primitives or subtasks. This is followed by recognition, modeling, and execution of the subtasks. LfD is particularly suited for complex surgical procedures; possibly the best way to transfer expert knowledge to the surgical robot.

Reinforcement learning: Reinforcement learning (RL) refers to the ability of an agent to learn the best possible action to be executed based on rewards obtained. Through iterative interaction with the environment, the agent accumulates rewards. Action that yields the highest reward is selected. Such a concept is utilized for deciphering the best optimal method to accomplish subtasks such as tube insertion and soft-tissue manipulation, when a complete, precise analytical model may not be available.[14] Real-time RL on a surgical robot is not feasible; simulations are performed to suitably train an RL agent. The trained agent is transferred to the real surgical robotic system. Reconciliation between real and simulated environment is a major challenge.

Augmented visualization and guidance: Effectively combining vision and touch sensors have improved the adaptability and intelligence of the surgical robot. 3D high-definition visualization of navigation path and the surgical site is made possible, together with high-resolution images of the texture and topography of the tissues. The aim is to achieve augmented reality; multi-modal visualization wherein 3D anatomical models are superimposed on live video feeds. Virtual reality (VR) coupled with such high-definition visualization is opening up new avenues; offering surgeons the perspective of being inside the patient. This would improve manifold, image-guided navigation and reduce cognitive load of a surgeon. Surgeries in difficult and otherwise obscured anatomy would be increasingly possible. Further, complete 3D mapping of the surgical site would provide opportunities for optimal planning leading to increased accuracy.

Tool-tissue interaction and haptics: Surgeons regularly use *haptics*, the sense of touch to navigate, detect tissues, and gauge forces. Current robotic surgical systems lack sufficient and accurate haptic feedback. Consequential feedback can be obtained from some estimation of the interaction forces between surgical tools and human tissues. AI techniques have been explored for and vision-based force and haptic feedback.

Human-machine interface: Surgical task-oriented HRIs have been explored through AI and ML techniques to control surgical robotic systems with touchless manipulation. Gaze, head movement, speech/voice, and hand gestures have been used. Human intent recognition is a challenge; appropriate solutions worked out exploiting AI allows the robot to perform the most appropriate action expected by the surgeon. This leads to perfect collaboration between the two. Further, AI and ML have started to be exploited for creating synergetic human-machine system comprising the surgeon and a surgical robot. This is based on efforts made elsewhere, particularly within rehabilitation robotics to develop neuroprostheses and bionic systems, linking the human musculoskeletal and nervous systems to external devices.[15] This requires decoding neural signals and establishing a feedback control loop via the peripheral nervous system.

Autonomous Surgical Robotics: The Future is Here

With a number of AI-enabled technologies endowing the surgical robot with intelligence, the next logical step is toward an autonomous surgical robot. Autonomy while manipulating soft-tissues is a difficult problem. Nevertheless, autonomous surgical robot is no longer science fiction. Numerous efforts have led to intelligent surgical robots with varying degrees of autonomy. Early tests results are promising. Many robotic systems are proving to be equals of surgeons, although at a miniscule of technical tasks.

Levels of autonomy: Autonomy achievable by a surgical robot has started to be taken seriously; and classified into six distinct levels.[16,17] Level 0 refers to no autonomy and level 5 referring to full autonomy; with intermediate levels of robot assistance, task autonomy, conditional autonomy and high autonomy. Most of the surgical robotic platforms available commercially are at level-0 and not autonomous. The motion of the robotic manipulator is under the exclusive control of the surgeon. Level-1 autonomy is about robotic assistance. No control is passed on to the robot; robotic assistance in terms of active constraints and virtual fixture is provided to the surgeon. For task autonomy under level-2, control switches from the human operator to the robot for the duration of the task to be executed. However, the robot is bereft of any ability to plan the task. Level-3 autonomy brings with its perceptual capabilities to not only understand surgical scenarios but also conceive strategies for optimal performance. However, any plan developed autonomously by the robot needs to be endorsed by the surgeon. Level-3 autonomy exploits many of the AI-enabled technologies enumerated earlier to sense, plan and act under supervision. Monitoring and plan updating is in real-time. For example, performance of a suturing task would involve the system extracting the suturing points and the length of each suture from real-time imaging, thereafter planning and executing the same. Level-4, i.e., high autonomy systems can interpret preoperative and intraoperative information, autonomously make clinical decisions. Execution is under constant supervision by the surgeon. Though sparingly, baby steps toward level-4 autonomy have been taken.[18] Level-5 indicates full autonomy where no human control is necessary. Such systems are still research ideation, but powered by AI and ML technologies definitely achievable. While there remain clear technical challenges, progress is hampered by ethical and regulatory aspects.

Early results have shown autonomous surgical robots to be equally good, if not better than the human counterpart, for many surgical maneuvers such as locating wounds, suturing, and removing tumors.[19] Assistance is destined to move to a next level; the robot would no longer remain a tool, rather it would become a surgical collaborator. This would hopefully allow the surgeon to focus on more complex decisions and undertake intricate surgical feats.

■ CONCLUSION

Robotic surgery is evolving at an unprecedented speed and penetrating a range of specialities. Microbots and autonomous surgical robotics are poised to emerge as the key enabling technologies. Newer robotic surgery systems are designed to be more precise with greater autonomy. Open-ended learning would open up further possibilities of autonomy.[20] As robotic surgical systems garner more autonomy, surgical performance and patient outcome promises to be improved. Novel functions would need to be added to such surgical systems. Surgical robotics would continue to draw inspiration from biological systems.

■ REFERENCES

1. Kwoh YS, Hou J, Jonckheere EA, Hayati S. A robot with improved absolute positioning accuracy for CT guided stereotactic brain surgery. IEEE Transact Biomed Engineer. 1988;35:153-60.
2. Ashrafian H, Clancy O, Grover V, Darzi A. The evolution of robotic surgery: surgical and anaesthetic aspects. BJA: Br JAnaesth. 2017;119(Suppl 1):i72-84.
3. Boyraz P, Dobrev I, Fischer G, Popovic MB. Robotic surgery. United States: Biomecatronics, Academic Press; 2019. pp. 431-50.
4. Khandalavala K, Shimon T, Flores L, Armijo PR, Oleynikov D. Emerging surgical robotic technology: a progression toward microbots. Ann Laparosc Endosc Surg. 2020;5:3.
5. Attanasio A, Scaglioni B, De Momi E, Fiorini P, Valdastri P. Autonomy in surgical robotics. Ann Rev Control Robotics Autonomous Syst. 2021;4:651-769.
6. Liu Y, Liu J. Surgical robotics: A look-back of latest advancement and bio-inspired ways to tackle existing challenges. Front Mech Engineer. 2012;7(4):376-84.
7. State of Art in Biomimetics Lepora NF, Verschure P, Prescott TJ. The state of the art in biomimetics. Bioinspir biomimet. 2013;8(1): 013001.
8. Malekzadeh MS, Calinon S, Bruno D, Caldwell DG. Learning by imitation with the STIFF-FLOP surgical robot: a biomimetic approach inspired by octopus movements. Robot Biomimet. 2014;1(1):1-5.
9. Li J, Esteban-Fernández de Ávila B, Gao W, Zhang L, Wang J. Micro/Nanorobots for Biomedicine: Delivery, Surgery, Sensing, and Detoxification. Sci Robot. 2017;2(4): eaam6431.
10. Ciuti G, Caliò R, Camboni D, Neri L, Bianchi F, Arezzo A, et al. Frontiers of robotic endoscopic capsules: a review. J microbio robot. 2016;11(1):1-8.
11. Palagi S, Fischer P. Bioinspired microrobots. Nat Rev Mater. 2018;3(6):113-24.

12. Leong TG, Randall CL, Benson BR, Bassik N, Stern GM, Gracias DH. Tetherless thermobiochemically actuated microgrippers. Proc Natl Acad Sci USA. 2009;106: 703-8.
13. Murali A, Sen S, Kehoe B, Garg A, McFarland S, Patil S, et al. Learning by observation for surgical subtasks: multilateral cutting of 3D viscoelastic and 2D orthotropic tissue phantoms. In: Zhou XY (Eds). Proceedings of IEEE International, 429 Conference on Robotics and Automation (ICRA). Seattle: IEEE; 2015. pp. 1202-9.
14. Kober J, Bagnell JA, Peters J. Reinforcement learning in robotics: a survey. Int J Robot Res. 2013;32(11):1238-74.
15. Basumatary H, Hazarika SM. State of the art in bionic hands. IEEE Transact Human-Machine Syst. 2020;50(2):116-30.
16. Dupont PE, Nelson BJ, Goldfarb M, Hannaford B, Menciassi A, O'Malley MK, et al. A decade retrospective of medical robotics research from 2010 to 2020. Sci Robot. 2021;6(60):eabi8017.
17. Yang GZ, Cambias J, Cleary K, Daimler E, Drake J, Dupont PE, et al. Medical robotics—Regulatory, ethical, and legal considerations for increasing levels of autonomy. Sci Robot. 2017;2(4):eaam8638.
18. Hu Y, Li W, Zhang L, Yang GZ. Designing, prototyping, and testing a flexible suturing robot for transanal endoscopic microsurgery. IEEE Robot Autom Lett. 2019;4(2):1669-75.
19. Fagogenis G, Mencattelli M, Machaidze Z, Rosa B, Price K, Wu F, et al. Autonomous robotic intracardiac catheter navigation using haptic vision. Sci Robot. 2019;4(29): eaaw1977.
20. Oddi A, Rasconi R, Santucci VG, Sartor G, Cartoni E, Mannella F, et al. (2020). Integrating open-ended learning in the sense-plan-act robot control paradigm. 24th European Conference on Artificial Intelligence—ECAI 2020. [online] Available from: chrome-extension://efaidnbmnnnibpcajpcglclefindmkaj/https://www.goal-robots.eu/wp-content/uploads/2021/06/2020_ODDI_ECAI_2020.pdf [Last accessed November, 2022].

Index

Page numbers followed by *b* refer to box, *f* refer to figure and *t* refer to table

A

Abdominal ports, placement of 82*f*
Accessory left hepatic artery 83*f*
Acinar cell cystadenoma 156
Adnexa, removal of 190*f*
American College of Surgeons Surgical Risk Calculator 53
American Society for Metabolic and Bariatric Surgery 171
American Society of Anesthesiologists Score 53
Anastomosis 52
Anastomotic leak 46, 52, 87
Anastomotic stenosis 87
Anesthesia 78
    perioperative management 113
Aorta, arch of 80*f*
Artificial intelligence 31, 37, 39, 41*f*, 46, 47, 47*f*-49*f*, 50*b*, 51*f*, 52, 54, 193, 194, 197
    development 43
    facets of 197
Artificial narrow intelligence 47
Artificial neural networks 48
Augmented visualization 198
Auris surgical robotics 13
Automated performance metrics 31
Automation 22
Autonomous surgical robotics 199
Autonomy, levels of 199
Avatera surgical system 8
Axesse equipment 15
Azygos vein bleeding 87

B

Bariatric surgery 169, 173
Barrett's esophagus 174
Bayesian linear regression 51
Bile duct injury 38
Biliopancreatic diversion 169, 173
Binocular stereoscopic 3D vision 73
Biomimetic micro-instruments 196
Biopsy forceps 125*f*, 150*f*
Bitrack system 7, 7*f*
Blood loss, estimated 98
Body mass index 171
Branch duct intraductal papillary mucinous neoplasia 158
British Association of Urological Surgeons modular pathways 28*f*
Bronchial artery, right 80*f*
Bronchoscopy systems 1

C

Calot's triangle 42
Camera, stability of 73
Cancer, rectal 96
Capsule endoscopy 16
Carbohydrate antigen 155
Carcinoembryonic antigen 155
Carcinoma 107
Centers for Disease Control and Prevention 114
Central pancreatectomy 160
Chemotherapy
    aerosolization of 126*f*
    intraperitoneal 120, 121
    neoadjuvant 77, 84
Cholecystectomy 37
Cholecystocaval line 150*f*
Circumferential radial margins 99
Clavien-Dindo classification 85
Colon cancer 96
Colorectal cancer 46, 52, 59, 64, 99
Colorectal lesions, endoscopic tattooing of 63
Colorectal surgery, current robotic systems for 97*t*
Colpotomy
    anterior 190*f*
    approach of 190*f*
    complete anterior 190*f*
Common bile duct 39*f*, 40*f*
Common hepatic artery 83*f*
    division of 147*f*
Competency assessment tool 26, 30

Index

Computed tomography 161
    imaging 2
    scan 49, 174
Contrast upper gastrointestinal study 174
Coronavirus disease 2019 (COVID-19)
    pandemic 113, 114
CUSUM chart 29*f*
Cyborgs 196
Cyst
    congenital 156
    endometrial 156
    enterogeneous 156
    retention 156
Cystadenocarcinoma, serous 156
Cystic acinar cell carcinoma 156
Cystic duct 39*f*
Cystic ductal adenocarcinoma 156
Cystic neuroendocrine tumor 156
Cystic pancreatoblastoma 156
Cytoreductive surgery 121

D

Da Vinci system 1, 20, 77, 96, 102, 185
    components of 2*f*
    docking of 111*f*
Deep learning 46, 47*f*
Deep vein thrombosis 87
Deoxyribonucleic acid 155
Dexter 8
Diaphragmatic hiatal hernia 87
Diode thulium: yttrium aluminum
    garnet 112
Distal pancreatectomy 162*f*
    operative technique for 161
Dual-docking techniques 138
Duodenal switch 173
Dysontogenetic cyst 156

E

EAU Robotic Urology Section
    curriculum 24*f*
Echocardiography 14
E-learning 24
Electrocardiogram 14
Electrode 126*f*
Electroprecipitation 126*f*
Embolism, pulmonary 87
Endoluminal surgery, robot
    capable of 12
Endomaster endoluminal access surgery
    efficacy system 13
Endoscopic biliary surgery, development
    of 37
Endoscopic robots 13
Endoscopic surgical systems 1
Endowrist instrumentation 73
Enucleation 160
Esophageal cancer, resectable 75
Esophagectomy 83*f*
    robot-assisted 75
Esophagitis 174
European Association of Endoscopic
    Surgery 20

F

Ferritin 171
Flex robotic system 9, 9*f*
Flexible carbon dioxide laser 112
Flexible robotic arms 10*f*
Flexible telescope 10*f*
Flexometallic tube 110
Fluorescence angiography 59, 61
Folate 171
Foley catheter 78
Freehand collaborative robot 15
Functional organ preservation surgery 107

G

Gastric
    banding, adjustable 169, 173
    conduit 83*f*, 84*f*
    emptying
        delayed 87
        studies 174
Gastroesophageal junction 83*f*
Gastroesophageal reflux
    disease 171, 173
Gastrointestinal oncology 120
Gastrointestinal origin 120
    peritoneal cancer of 129*t*
Gastrointestinal surgery 138
Gastrointestinal tumors 13
Gastroplasty, vertical banded 169
Gastrostomy supplementation 109
Global assessment scale tools 26, 29

H

Harmonic robotic arm, option of 73
Harmonic scalpel 150*f*
Hemogram, complete 171
Hepatic artery 147*f*
    right 148*f*

Index

Hepatic duct, division of 148*f*
Hepatic hilum, dissection of 146
Hepatic left medial segment,
    lower edge of 39*f*
Hepatic transection 150*f*
Hepatic vein 149*f*
Hepatobiliary surgery,
    robot-assisted 145
Hepatocaval dissection 147
High-resolution manometry 174
Hinotori robotic
    system 3, 4*f*
    platform 11*f*
Hominis surgical system 10
Hugo® RAS system 4
Human papillomavirus 109, 115
Hydrogel polyvinyl alcohol 25
Hyperthermic intraperitoneal
    chemotherapy 121
Hypopharyngeal lesions 109
Hysterectomy, laparoscopic 185

I

Index bariatric operation 172*t*
Index bariatric procedure
    complications of 171
    failure of 170
Indocyanine green 60, 82, 147
    fluorescence 62*f*, 66
        angiography 60, 63
        system 61*f*
    injection 84*f*
    properties of 60
Information-rich platform
    development 40*f*
Instruments fenestrated bipolar hot shears,
    selection of 185*f*
Intensive care unit 76
Intraductal papillary mucinous
    neoplasm 153, 156
Intraperitoneal catheter 121
Intravascular compartment 61*f*
Invendoscopy E210 system 13
Iris technology 2
Iron profile 171

L

Lap mentor equipment 15
Laparoendoscopic single
    port surgery 194
    site surgical systems 1, 9

Laparoscopic
    assisted surgery 99
    cholecystectomy 37, 41*f*
        anatomical landmarks for 39*f*
    distal pancreatectomy 162*f*
    hysterectomy, robot-assisted 185
    intraoperative ultrasonography,
        use of 162*f*
    partial nephrectomy,
        robot-assisted 27*f*
    peritoneal biopsy 125*f*
    pyeloplasty, robot-assisted 27*f*
    ventral mesh rectopexy 101
Large cystic tumor 162*f*
Laryngeal nerve injury, recurrent 87
Learning curve 23, 74, 177
Left gastric artery 83*f*
Left recurrent laryngeal nerve 81*f*
Lesser omentum 83*f*
Linear regression 51
Liquid chemotherapy 123*f*
Liver
    demarcation of 150*f*
    function test 171
    resection, robot-assisted 145,
        146, 149
    transection of 149
Lymph node 98
    median numbers of 86
Lymphoepithelial cyst 156

M

Machine learning 46, 47*f*, 48, 49*f*, 53*f*
    types of 50
Magnetic resonance imaging 48
Malformation syndromes 156
Mammography 49
Mazor robotics' renaissance 14
Medical microinstruments symani robotic
    microsurgery system 14
Micro hand S 6
    surgical system 7*f*
Micro-electro-mechanical
    systems 197
Micromate robot 15
Micro-pump 126*f*
    midline installation of 126*f*
Micro-robotic procedures 195
Miliary peritoneal carcinosis 124*f*
Miniaturized in vivo robotic assistant
    surgical robot platform 12*f*
    virtual incision miniature robot 11
Minimal access surgery 96

Index

Minimally invasive
   distal pancreatic resection 163
   esophagectomy 72
      robot-assisted 72
   liver resection 145
   pancreatic surgery 153
      current status of 153
   surgery 20, 74, 145, 193
      learning curve of 74f
   techniques 72
Monarch 13
Monopolar
   hook 125f
   scissors 185f
Morrison's pouch 149
Mucinous cystic neoplasm 153, 156, 158
Mucinous non-neoplastic cyst 156
Multicenter randomized controlled
      trials 115

N

Naïve Bayes classifier 51
Nathanson's retractor 161
National Institute for Health and Care
      Excellence 26, 107
National Training Programme for
      Laparoscopic Colorectal
      Surgery 26
Natural orifice transluminal endoscopic
      surgery 15, 194
Near-infrared perfusion index 66
Negative-pressure otolaryngology viral
      isolation drape 114
Nodal dissection 81f

O

Observational clinical human reliability
      analysis 30
Obstructive sleep apnea 171
One-anastomosis gastric bypass 169, 173
Open console systems 3
Open esophagectomy 71
Open surgery 98
Open three-dimensional console
      systems 1
Open transthoracic esophagectomy 72, 75
Operating room set-up 178, 178f
Operation
   tables 4
   technique 78
Operative system 77

Organ prolapse repair 100
Ovarian ligament 186f

P

Pancreas, superior border of 83f
Pancreatic cystic neoplasms 153, 154t, 158
   classification of 156b
Pancreaticoduodenectomy 156
Parenchyma sparing procedures 159
   operative technique for 163
Periampullary duodenal wall cyst 156
Peritoneal cancer 120, 129t, 131t
Peritoneal carcinomatics cancer 120
Peritoneal carcinomatosis 120
   index 124f
Peritoneal regression grading score 131, 131t
Peritoneal washing cytology 124f
Peritonectomy 125f
   edges, demarcation of 125f
Peritoneum, uterovesical fold of 187f
Pfannenstiel incision 149
Pleural effusion 87
Pneumonia 87
Port placement 179, 186
Port positions 141f, 146f
Portal vein 163
Positron emission tomography scans 49
Postoperative pancreatic fistula 156
Post-therapeutic organ dysfunction 109
Povidone-iodine 114
Powerspiral enteroscope 16
Precision surgery 59
Pressurized intraperitoneal aerosol
      chemotherapy 120, 121,
      123f, 129t
   procedure technique 120, 122
Prolapse, rectal 96
Proximal pancreatic division 162f
Pulmonary artery bleeding 87
Pure endoscopy 1

R

Radical prostatectomy,
   robot assisted 3, 27f
Recurrent nasopharyngeal cancer after
      radiotherapy 109
Reinforcement learning 51, 198
Renal function test 171
Renin angiotensin system 113
Reoperative bariatric surgery 175
   indications of 170

Index

Retraction robot 15
Revisional bariatric surgery, robot assisted 169, 176, 177, 179*f*
Right hepatic vein 149*f*
   division of 148*f*
   intra-capsular control of 150*f*
Right subclavian artery 80*f*
Right vaginal vault angle 190*f*
Robotic
   anterior resection, port positions for 99*f*
   bariatric surgery 138
   colorectal surgery 96
   console skills, assessment of 30
   distal pancreatectomy 162*f*
   endoscopy systems 1
   esophageal resections 71
   esophagectomy 73, 74, 74*f*, 84
   hepatectomy 145
   hysterectomy 185
   minimal access surgical systems 1
   natural orifice transluminal endoscopic surgery 107
   platform 108
   rectal cancer
      studies 97*t*
      surgery 96
   right colectomy 101
   skills, global evaluation assessment of 30
   stapler 141*f*
   summative assessment tools 30
   surgery 21, 30, 98, 138, 142, 153, 193, 197
      assessment 20
      automated assessment tools in 31
      cost analysis of 102
      fundamentals of 22
      training 20
   system 97
   telementoring 102
   training curricula 22
   transoral surgery 107
   ventral mesh rectopexy 100, 101
      port positions of 101*f*
Rouviere's sulcus 38, 39*f*
Roux-en-Y gastric bypass 169, 173
   surgery 138

S

Sacral promontory 101*f*
Salsa
   maneuver 188
   technique 188*f*
Scorpion-shaped endoscopic robot 15
Sensei X robotic catheter system 14
Sentinel lymph node mapping 64
Serous cystic neoplasm 153, 156, 158
Serum iron 171
Severe acute respiratory syndrome coronavirus 2 113
Single port systems 1
Sinha-Apollo technique 185
Sleeve gastrectomy 169, 173
Snow storm 126*f*
Sole biopsy 52
Solid pseudopapillary neoplasm 153, 156, 158
Spleen 162*f*
Stereoscopic surgeon console systems 1
Stoma 52
Superior mesenteric vein 163
Support vector machines 51
Surgery 193
   laparoscopic 98
   system, robot assisted 5*f*, 194
Symani robotic microsurgery system 14*f*

T

Thoracic duct 80*f*
   injury 87
Thoracic esophagectomy, operative steps of 80*f*
Tissue
   optical window 60
   oxygen saturation 66
   water index 66
Total mesorectal excision 96, 98, 99*f*
Trachea, membranous part of 81*f*
Transferrin saturation 171
Transhiatal esophagectomy, robot assisted 73
Transoral oropharyngeal defects, classification system for 107
Transoral robotic
   reconstruction surgery 107
   sleep apnea 107
   surgery 107, 109, 110*f*, 111*f*, 112
      advantage of 112*b*
      benefit of 112
      complications of 113
      pearls of 110
   thyroidectomy 107
   total laryngectomy 109
Trendelenburg's position 161
Trocar placement 146

U

Ultrasounds 49
Ureter visualization 63
Urology procedures 138
Uterine artery coagulation
        transection 188*f*
Uterosacral ligaments 187*f*

V

Vaginal vault suturing 191*f*
Vena cava
    inferior 147
    superior 80*f*
Versius robotic system 5*f*

Vicarious surgical miniature robot 11
Video-assisted thoracoscopic surgery 73
Vocal cord palsy 87
von Hippel-Lindau 155

W

Warshaw's technique 163
Weight loss
    excess 170
    insufficient 170
Wound infection 87

X

XACT ace robotic system 15